D0098952

i'll start again monday

Other Books and DVD Bible Studies by Lysa

i'll start again monday

BREAK THE CYCLE OF UNHEALTHY EATING
HABITS WITH LASTING SPIRITUAL SATISFACTION

LYSA TERKEURST

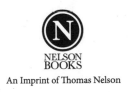

NELSON
BOOKS

An Imprint of Thomas Nelson

I'll Start Again Monday

© 2022 Lysa TerKeurst

Abridged from *Made to Crave*, 9780310293262, © 2010.

Published in Nashville, Tennessee, by Nelson Books, an imprint of Thomas Nelson. Nelson Books and Thomas Nelson are registered trademarks of HarperCollins Christian Publishing, Inc.

Thomas Nelson titles may be purchased in bulk for educational, business, fundraising, or sales promotional use. For information, please e-mail SpecialMarkets@ThomasNelson.com.

Unless otherwise noted, Scripture quotations are from The Holy Bible, New International Version®, NIV®. Copyright © 1973, 1978, 1984, 2011 by Biblica, Inc.® Used by permission of Zondervan. All rights reserved worldwide. www.Zondervan.com. The "NIV" and "New International Version" are trademarks registered in the United States Patent and Trademark Office by Biblica, Inc.®

Scripture quotations marked NASB are from New American Standard Bible®. Copyright © 1960, 1962, 1963, 1968, 1971, 1972, 1973, 1975, 1977, 1995 by The Lockman Foundation. Used by permission. (www.Lockman.org)

Scripture quotations marked NLT are from the Holy Bible, New Living Translation. © 1996, 2004, 2007, 2013, 2015 by Tyndale House Foundation. Used by permission of Tyndale House Publishers, Inc., Carol Stream, Illinois 60188. All rights reserved.

Any internet addresses, phone numbers, or company or product information printed in this book are offered as a resource and are not intended in any way to be or to imply an endorsement by Thomas Nelson, nor does Thomas Nelson vouch for the existence, content, or services of these sites, phone numbers, companies, or products beyond the life of this book.

ISBN 978-0-7852-3250-6 (eBook)
ISBN 978-0-7852-3248-3 (HC)

Library of Congress Control Number: 2021945798

Printed in the United States of America

22 23 24 25 26 LSC 10 9 8 7 6 5

To the girl with a weary heart who feels so very alone in this struggle that seems like it will never end . . . Let me be the friend who comes alongside you to say: you are seen. You are loved. You are prayed for. Jesus is with you, and so am I. We can do this. So, let's link arms and face this journey together.

contents

introduction

Finding Your "Want To"

A typical book on healthy lifestyle choices should contain lots of talk on vegetables, calories, colon cleanses, and phrases like "you must" and "you should."

I have a problem with all that talk. It's not the "how to" I'm missing. It's the "want to" ... really wanting to make lasting changes and deciding that the results of those changes are worth the sacrifice.

In light of this admission, I think it's only appropriate to be honest with you about a few things right up front.

1. I am emotionally allergic to typical books on healthy eating.
2. Not once in my life have I ever craved a carrot stick.
3. I am not overly excited about giving up two of the greatest delights of my taste buds—Cheez-Its and box-mix brownies. In fact, I've asked God if it would be such a terribly difficult thing to swap the molecular structure of Cheez-Its for carrot

sticks. They're both already orange. And, really, how hard could that be for someone who's turned water into wine?

4. I wasn't sure I had any business writing a book like this. I'm a simple Jesus girl on a journey to finding deeper motivation than just a number on my scale for getting and staying healthy.

I'm not writing this book to beat your taste buds into submission or because I've discovered the magic diet to get you skinny by tomorrow. I'm writing this book because I've struggled way too long with my food choices and my weight. Because I've said, "I'll start again Monday" a thousand times—only to disappoint myself by breakfast. And word on the street says most of my girlfriends fight this draining, dissatisfying cycle day in and day out as well. Which brings me to the fifth thing you should know about me:

5. I started this journey weighing 167 pounds. To some, this is a horrifyingly high number. To others, 167 is a dream weight. In my case, the number itself was not the issue. The issue was how I felt mentally, spiritually, and physically. It was time to be honest with myself.

I think we all get to a place in our lives when we have to give a brutally honest answer to the question, "How am I doing?" It's not really a conversation we have with a friend or family member. It's one of those middle-of-the-night contemplations when there's no glossing over the realities staring us in the face.

I knew certain things about myself needed to change, but it was easier to make excuses than it was to tackle them head-on. Rationalizations are so appealing. See if you relate to any of these:

> *I'm good in every other area.*
> *I make so many sacrifices already.*
> *I need treats as a comfort in this season of life; I'll deal with my issues later.*
> *The Bible doesn't specifically say this is wrong.*
> *If I really wanted to make a change, I could; I just don't want to right now.*
> *Oh, for heaven's sake, everyone has issues. So what if this is mine?*

But excuses got me nowhere fast, especially when it came to healthy eating.

A whole lifetime could be spent giving in to excuses, feeling guilty, resolving to do better, mentally beating myself up for not sticking to my resolve, and then resigning myself to the fact that things can't change.

And I don't want to spend a lifetime in this cycle.

I suspect you don't either.

The book you hold in your hands could be the missing companion you've needed with every healthy eating plan you tried and cried over. I believe it will help you find your "want to."

In addition to helping you find the desire to conquer your unhealthy eating habits, it also holds the key to something very significant for most of us women: spiritual malnutrition. We feel overweight physically but underweight spiritually. Tying these two things together is the first step on one of the most significant journeys you'll ever take with God.

It reminds me of a journey described in Matthew 19. A rich young man comes to see Jesus and explains that he is following all the rules but still feels something missing from his pursuit of God. "All these [rules] I have kept," he says. "What do I still lack?" (v. 20). Or, in other words, "I'm doing the basics of what's required . . . so why do I still feel that I'm missing something?"

Such a vulnerable question. Such a relatable question.

Jesus responds, "If you want to be perfect [whole], go, sell your possessions and give to the poor, and you will have treasure in heaven. Then come, follow me" (v. 21).

The rich young man then goes away sad because he won't give up the one thing that consumes him. He is so full with his riches he can't see how undernourished his soul is. He's just like people today who refuse egg whites and fruit for breakfast so they can fill themselves up with candy-sprinkled, chocolate-frosted doughnuts. Even when their sugar high crashes and they complain of splitting headaches, they steadfastly refuse to give up their doughnuts.

In my past sugar-filled life, I might have had some personal experience that led me to think of that frail little analogy.

Anyhow.

Jesus didn't mean this as a sweeping command for everyone who has a lot of money. He meant this for any of us who wallow in whatever abundance we have. I imagine Jesus looked straight into this young man's soul and said, "I want you to give up the one thing you crave more than me. Then come, follow me."

Piercing thought, isn't it?

Suddenly, Jesus isn't just staring at the rich young man; He's also staring at me—the inside me. The part I can't cover up with excuses and makeup.

When Jesus wants us to follow Him—really follow Him—it's serious business: "If anyone wants to come after Me, he must deny himself, take up his cross, and follow Me" (Mark 8:34 NASB).

With Jesus, if we want to gain, we must give up.

To be filled, we must deny ourselves.

To truly get close to God, we'll have to distance ourselves from other things.

To conquer our cravings, we'll have to redirect them to God.

God made us capable of craving so we'd have an unquenchable desire for more of Him, and Him alone.

Nothing changes until we make the choice to redirect our misguided cravings to the only One capable of satisfying them.

Getting healthy isn't just about losing weight. It's about recalibrating our souls so that we want to change—spiritually, physically, and mentally. And the battle really is in all three areas.

Spiritually. I had to ask God to give me the desire to be healthy. I knew a vanity-seeking "want to" would never last. Shallow desires produce only shallow efforts. I had to seek a spiritual "want to" empowered by God Himself.

So, I asked. I begged, actually. I cried out to God. And day by day, God gave me just enough "want to," laced with His strength, to be satisfied by healthy choices.

God also settled in my heart that this is an issue of great spiritual importance. Think of Eve in the Bible's first recorded interaction between a woman and food. Obviously, the core of Eve's temptation was that she wanted to be like God, knowing good and evil. But we can't ignore the fact that *the serpent used food as a tool in the process.* If the very downfall of humanity was caused when Eve surrendered to a temptation to eat something she wasn't supposed to eat, I do think our struggles with food are important to God.

Physically. The spiritual perspectives in this book may stir the soul, but the physical realities require turning those spiritual insights into practical choices.

When I began this journey, I finally had to admit

that what I eat matters. My weight is a direct reflection of my choices and the state of my health.

I started with a visit to my doctor, which I highly encourage you to do before starting your healthy eating plan. The doctor ran several tests. Except for some results that indicated I wasn't exercising regularly or making the healthiest food choices, the tests came back normal.

Hmfff. Why do doctors always say the same old thing about eating right and exercise?

Feeling sluggish? Eat better, move more. Feeling blue? Eat better, move more. I bet the next time I go in for a sore throat it will be the same thing. Eat better, move more. Have mercy. And we won't even go into the issues I have with the scale in my doctor's office. I am positive it weighs me heavy just to prove his point. *See? You need to eat better, move more.*

The doctor and the test results were right. My weight issues were directly linked to my food choices. Period. I had to admit it and do something about it.

Mentally. I had to decide I was tired of compromising. What happens when you delete "com" from the word *compromise*? You're left with a "promise." We were made for more than *compromise.* We were made for God's *promises* in every area of our lives.

Honestly, I am made for more than a vicious cycle of eating, gaining, stressing—eating, gaining, stressing . . . I am made to rise up, do battle with my issues, and, using the Lord's strength in me, defeat them to the glory of God.

I hope you'll stick around on this journey of discovering your "want to." I can't promise it will be easy. But I can promise it will be the most empowering thing you've ever done. Just today I put on some jeans I never thought I'd wear again. And while my flesh did the happy dance of success, my soul was far from thoughts of vanity.

My soul felt free. I was amazed that I ever desired to satisfy my taste buds over satisfying my desire to break free from all the guilt, all the destruction, all the defeat.

I still don't crave those blasted carrot sticks. But I found my "want to." I started eating better and moving more. I lost the weight. I feel great. And I have most certainly grown closer to God than ever before.

My truest cravings are satisfied—and yours can be too.

what's really going on here?

Several years ago, a weight-loss company came up with a brilliant advertising campaign. Maybe you saw some of their ads. A little orange monster chases a woman around, tempting and taunting her with foods that obviously aren't a part of her healthy eating plan. The ads perfectly captured what it feels like to be harassed by cravings all day long.

While the orange monster is a great way to visualize cravings, the ads fall short in their promise to really help a woman. The weight-loss company's theory is to teach what foods are more filling and encourage consumption of those. But does that really help overcome cravings?

For me, it does not. Simply telling me to eat healthier foods that will help me feel full longer doesn't address the heart of the matter. I can feel full after a meal and still crave chocolate pie for dessert. Just feeling full isn't the answer to sticking with a healthy eating plan.

So, what's really going on here?

I believe God made us to crave. Now before you think this is some sort of cruel joke by God, let me assure you that the object of our craving was never supposed to be food or other things people find themselves consumed by, such as sex or money or chasing after significance.

Think about the definition of the word *craving*. Dictionary.com defines *craving* as "something you long for, want greatly, desire eagerly, and beg for."[1] Now consider this expression of craving: "How lovely is your dwelling place, Lord Almighty! My soul yearns, even faints, for the courts of the Lord; my heart and my flesh cry out for the living God" (Psalm 84:1–2).

Yes, we were made to crave—long for, want greatly, desire eagerly, and beg for—God. Only God. But Satan wants to replace our craving for God with something else. Here's what the Bible says about this: "Do not love the world or anything in the world. . . . For everything in the world—the cravings of sinful man, the lust of his eyes and the boasting of what he has and does—comes not from the Father but from the world" (1 John 2:15–16).

The passage details three ways Satan tries to lure us away from loving God:

- The cravings of the sinful man
- The lust of his eyes
- The boasting of what he has or does

Let's define these things.

According to the commentary in my *Life Application Study Bible* (NIV):

Cravings = trying to get our physical desires met
   outside the will of God
Lust of eyes = trying to get our material desires met
   outside the will of God
Boasting = trying to get our need for significance
   met *outside the will of God*

Remember Eve? Studying her story, I realized how intentionally Satan chooses his tactics. He knows where we are weak. He desires to lure us away from God. And he knows what works . . . "When the woman saw that the fruit of the tree was good for food [cravings of the sinful man] and pleasing to the eye [lust of the eyes], and also desirable for gaining wisdom [boasting of what she has or does], she took some and ate it" (Genesis 3:6). Eve was tempted in precisely the same three ways the 1 John passage warns us about.

But it doesn't stop there. Look at how Jesus was tempted:

Then Jesus was led by the Spirit into the wilderness to be tempted by the devil. After fasting forty days and forty nights, he was hungry. The tempter came to him and said, "If you are the Son of God, tell these stones to become bread."

Jesus answered, "It is written: 'Man does not live on bread alone, but on every word that comes from the mouth of God.'"

Then the devil took him to the holy city and had him stand on the highest point of the temple. "If you are the Son of God," he said, "throw yourself down. For it is written:

> "'He will command his angels
>   concerning you,
> and they will lift you up in their hands,
>   so that you will not strike your
>   foot against a stone.'"

Jesus answered him, "It is also written: 'Do not put the Lord your God to the test.'"

Again, the devil took him to a very high mountain and showed him all the kingdoms of the world and their splendor. "All this I will give you," he said, "if you will bow down and worship me."

Jesus said to him, "Away from me, Satan! For it is written: 'Worship the Lord your God, and serve him only.'"

Then the devil left him, and angels came and attended him. (Matthew 4:1–11)

Again, the pattern of temptation is the same:

Cravings: Satan appealed to Jesus' physical cravings
for food.

Lust of the eyes: The devil promised Jesus entire
kingdoms if He would bow down to the god of
materialism.

Boasting: The enemy enticed Jesus to prove His
significance by forcing God to command
angels to save Him.

But here's the significant difference between Eve and
Jesus. Eve was saturated with the object of her desire. Jesus
was saturated with God's truth.

I obviously wasn't in the garden with Eve, but based
on three phrases from Genesis 3:6, I can only infer that
she never took her eyes off the fruit as she *saw that the
food was good, pleasing to the eye, and desirable.* She didn't
walk away and give herself time to consider her choice. She
didn't consult Adam. She didn't consider the truth of what
God had clearly instructed or talk to Him. She focused
only on the object of her obsession.

Eve craved what she focused on. We consume what
we think about. And what we think about can consume
us if we're not careful.

We crave what we eat. If I make healthy choices over
a period of time, it seems to reprogram my taste buds.
The more veggies and fruit I eat, the more veggies and

e. However, if I eat brownies and chips, I crave
___ ind chips in the worst kind of way.

Jesus set a beautiful example of breaking this vicious
cycle of being consumed by cravings. It's even more powerful when we understand that Jesus was in a completely
deprived state.

Eve was in a paradise garden with her every need provided for. Jesus had been in a wilderness, fasting for forty
days. And yet He held strong. He quoted God's Word.
And so can we. When we feel deprived and frustrated and
consumed with wanting unhealthy choices, we, too, can
rely on God's Word to help us.

With each temptation, Jesus quoted Scripture that
refuted Satan's temptation. Truth is powerful. The more
saturated we are with truth, the more powerful we'll be
in resisting our temptations. And the more we'll naturally
direct our cravings where they should be directed—to the
Author of all truth.

Cravings. Are they a curse or a blessing? The answer
to that depends on what we're craving. And what we're
craving will always depend on whatever we're consuming . . . the object of our desire or God and His truth.

Consider what it means to the success of your journey
to quote Scripture in the midst of a craving attack. One
of the most meaningful scriptures I used in this process is
" 'Everything is permissible'—but not everything is beneficial" (1 Corinthians 10:23). I quoted this scripture over
and over to remind myself that I could have that brownie

or those chips, but they wouldn't benefit me in any way. That thought empowered me to make a beneficial choice rather than wallowing in being deprived of an unhealthy choice. As you read this book, make a point to write out meaningful verses and quote them aloud each time the orange monster tries to talk you into tarrying with him awhile.

I know it's a battle, sister. But we aren't rendered powerless. The more saturated we are with God's truth, the more powerfully resistant we become. Stick with me here—this isn't a plastic Christian answer. It's one that will change our lives if we let it.

replacing my cravings

I roll over and look at the clock. Another day. Beyond all reason and rationality, I slide out of bed and strip off everything that might weigh even the slightest ounce as I head to the scale. Maybe today will be the day the scale will be my friend and not reveal my secrets. Maybe somehow overnight the molecular structure of my body shifted and today I will magically weigh less.

But no. I yank out my ponytail holder—hey, it's gotta weigh something—and decide to try again. But the scale doesn't change its mind the second time. It is not my friend this day.

Vowing to do better, eat healthier, and make good choices, I head to the kitchen only to have my resolve melt like the icing on the cinnamon rolls my daughter just pulled from the oven. Yum. Oh, who cares what the scale says when this roll speaks such love and deliciousness.

Two and a half cinnamon rolls later, I decide tomorrow will be a much better day to keep my promises to eat healthier. And since this is my last day to eat what I want, I better live it up. Another cinnamon roll, please.

The next morning I turn over and look at the clock. Another day. Beyond all reason and rationality, I slide out of bed and strip off everything that might weigh even the slightest ounce as I head to the scale. Maybe today will be the day. But once again it isn't. I yank out my ponytail holder and try again. But no.

Vowing to do better, eat healthier, and make good choices, I head into my day, only to find myself making more excuses, rationalizations, and promises for later.

Always later.

And the cycle I've come to hate and feel powerless to stop continues.

Who could I talk to about this? If I admit my struggle to my friends, they might try to hold me accountable the next time we go out. And what if I'm not in the mood to be questioned about my nachos con queso with extra sour cream? I'll just tell them I'll be starting on Monday, and they'll be fine with it. They don't think I need to make changes.

But I did need to make changes. I knew it. Because this wasn't really about the scale; it was about this battle that raged in my heart. I thought about, craved, and arranged my life too much around food. So much so, I knew it was something God was challenging me to surrender to His control. Really surrender. To the point where I'd make radical changes for the sake of my spiritual health perhaps even more than my physical health.

Part of my surrender was asking myself a really raw question.

May I ask you this same raw question?

Is it possible we love and rely on food more than we love and rely on God?

Now, before you throw this book across the room, hear me out. This question is crucial. I had to see the purpose of my struggle as something more than wearing smaller sizes and getting compliments from others.

It had to be about something more than just me.

I had to get honest enough to admit I relied on food more than I relied on God. Food was my comfort. My reward. My joy. Food was what I turned to in times of stress, sadness, and even in times of happiness.

I felt stupid admitting that. I felt like such a spiritual failure.

I told a few people about it and most seemed support-ive. But one well-meaning woman quipped what others would echo in the months that followed: "You're making this diet thing a spiritual journey? Does God really care about our food?"

Yes, I think He does.

God never intended for us to want anything more than we want Him. Just the slightest glimpse into His Word proves that. Look at what the Bible says when God's chosen people, the Israelites, wanted food more than they wanted God: "They willfully put God to the test by demanding the food they craved" (Psalm 78:18). Yikes.

And what became of them? They never reached the promised land. These people wandered in the desert for forty years, and no one but Joshua and Caleb (the ↑ generation leaders) was allowed to enter the land flowing with milk and honey.

I don't know about you, but I don't want to wander about in a "desert," unable to enter into the abundant life God has for me because I willfully put Him to the test over food!

When I started, I knew this battle would be hard. But through it all I determined to make God my focus. Each time I craved something I knew wasn't part of my plan, I used that craving as a prompt to pray. I craved a lot. So, I found myself praying a lot.

Don't rush past that last paragraph. I used my cravings for food as a prompting to pray. It was my way of tearing down the tower of impossibility before me and building something new. My tower of impossibility was food. Brick by brick, I imagined myself dismantling the food tower and using those same bricks to build a walkway of prayer, paving the way to victory.

Did this simple visualization make it easier? Sometimes it did. Other times my cravings for unhealthy food made me cry. Seriously, cry. Sometimes I wound up on the floor in my closet, praying with tears running down my face. And I gave myself permission to cry, just like the psalmist:

> Listen to my words, Lord,
>   consider my lament.
> Hear my cry for help,

---

my King and my God,
for to you I pray.
In the morning, LORD, you hear my
voice;
in the morning I lay my requests
before you
and wait expectantly.

(Psalm 5:1–3)

That is exactly what I did.

"God, I want a biscuit this morning. Instead, I'm eating poached eggs. I'm thankful for these eggs, but I'll be honest in saying my cravings for other things are hard to resist. But, instead of wallowing in what I *can't* have, I'm making the choice to celebrate what I *can* have."

"God, it's 10:00 a.m. and I'm craving again. I want those snack crackers that are screaming my name. But instead of reaching for them, I'm praying. I'll be honest, I don't want to pray. I want those crackers. But I'll have a handful of almonds and brick by brick . . . prayer by prayer . . . lay a path for victory."

"God, it's lunchtime and all my friends are heading out for Mexican. I love Mexican! I could seriously justify a big bowl of chips and guacamole right now. But once again I'm choosing to pray instead of getting stuck in my craving. Help me, God, to feel satisfied with healthier choices."

And that's how my prayers continued throughout

the day. Laying my requests before God and waiting in expectation.

Then one morning, it finally happened. I got up, and for the first time in a long while, I felt incredibly empowered. I still did the same crazy routine with the scale—no clothes, no ponytail holder—but I only stepped on it once. The numbers hadn't changed yet, but my heart had. One day of victory tasted better than any of that food I'd given up ever could. I had waited in expectation using prayer as my guide, and I did it.

I did it that day and the next. Then the next. Why not shoot for four victorious days in a row? And then maybe one more.

I can't promise you there won't be any more tears. And I can't promise the scale will magically drop as quickly as you wish it would. But it will be a start. A really good start.

getting a plan

Last spring I took a shortcut through a neighborhood and caught a glimpse of a man planting a flower garden. That quick glance was long enough to produce a lingering thought: *I wish I had a pretty garden.*

For years I've looked at other people's flowers and secretly wished for my own lush display. However, the glimpse of this man with his hands digging deep into the earth brought a new revelation. *He has a garden because he invests time and energy to make it.* He didn't wish it into being. He didn't just wake up one day and find that a garden of glorious blooms had miraculously popped up from the dirt.

No.

He worked at it. He sacrificed for it. Day after day. Row by row. Seed by seed. Plant by plant.

It took time and commitment before he ever saw any fruit from his labor. But eventually there was a bloom . . . and then another . . . and then another.

I saw this man's flowers and wished for my own—without a clue about all the work that had gone into producing them. I want the flowers but not the work.

Isn't that the way it is with many things in life—we want the results but have no desire to put in the work?

Besides a garden, I also wished for a thinner body for years but was lax about actually changing what I ate. I excused away the necessary discipline, citing my age and metabolism, lamenting the unfairness of my genetic disposition and blah, blah, blah.

The reality is, I can't eat like an athletic teenager and then complain about my extra layers of fluff.

Or my pants size.

Or my arms that are starting to wave back at me when I raise them.

I can't wish blooms into place any more than I can wish fat away. I knew I needed a plan. Something more than "I'll start again Monday."

I had a friend who'd found a nutritionist she really liked. She got her issues under control, lost weight, kept it off, and experienced the empowering feeling of success.

The day of my first appointment with this same nutritionist, I sat in my car and chuckled at my choice for a *last meal*—the meal before I'd have to make changes.

I stared down at the paper plate. Minutes before, it had been piled high with slices of Chef Boyardee pizza. Cheap, boxed pizza had been the delight of my childhood taste buds. Who am I kidding? It was the delight of my adulthood as well. And if my food choice alone didn't seal the deal that changes needed to be made, my next move certainly did.

I licked the plate.

Yes, I did. If this would be the last time I'd enjoy this delicacy, I was for sure not leaving a drop of sauce on the plate. Not a drop.

Inside the nutritionist's office, I was told I was overweight. This was not news to me. I had gone up two pants sizes during the past year and now even my big pants were protesting.

Something had to give.

Someone had to learn the discipline of giving up some things. And those "things" were poor food choices that were sabotaging my body, my mental energy, and my spirit.

Food had become like a drug. And honestly, it's a good drug choice for a Christian woman. Every church event I attended readily provided my drug out in the open with no hesitation or judgment.

I was eating too much of the wrong kinds of foods and felt trapped in a cycle of hunger. I felt hungry all the time. I was too dependent on food for comfort. I wanted to eat what I wanted, when I wanted, in the quantities I wanted. So, despite exercising, my food choices caught up with me, and my changing body revealed all my secrets.

That's both the blessing and the curse of issues with food. My poor choices will rat me out every time—if not in my waistline, then in my energy level and my overall well-being.

I left the nutritionist's office that day with a plan. Under her supervision and with a weekly weigh-in to hold me accountable, I felt empowered for the first time in a long while.

The plan I chose was strict and restrictive. I knew in my heart it had to be. I had to break the addictive cycles my taste buds had grown to crave. I needed to train my body not to be hungry all the time. I had to keep my blood sugar in check.

The healthy eating plan I adopted then and maintain now is a balanced protein-carbohydrate plan. I learned correct portion sizes, food combining, when to eat, and what to eat. I still eat carbohydrates, but I'm limited in how much and what kind. I don't eat most breads, potatoes, rice, corn, pasta, or other starchy things. Mainly, I eat low-fat meats, veggies, and fruits.

I have a funny truth to share about the healthy eating plan I chose. Basically, I eat what a wild animal eats— meat and things that grow naturally from the earth. Only I cook my food and use manners. I was immediately encouraged by the possibilities of this plan because I have yet to see an overweight animal in the wild lamenting over excess cellulite.

Think about it.

I'm not saying this has to be your plan. (You need to do your research, consult your doctor, and create a healthy and realistic plan for *your* everyday life.) I'm saying this is *my* plan and, believe it or not, I've grown to love it. Notice

I said "*grown* to love it." I won't deny there have been some really hard days.

My plan is realistic for me because the foods I eat are things I can buy at my local grocery store and because my family can eat what I eat for the most part. However, they usually have starches that I skip.

This journey will require you to make some tough sacrifices, but I've come to look at this process as embracing healthy choices rather than denying myself. There are lessons to be learned and perspectives to be gained in the season of embracing healthy choices. These will not just be physical lessons. The mental and spiritual lessons gained in this time will be the very thing to equip you for the long haul. And keep you healthy and blossoming, just like that man's garden.

Speaking of gardens, don't be expecting any fresh-cut flowers from my garden. That is still but a wish.

A girl can't do it all, you know.

friends don't let friends eat before thinking

Stop, in the name of love, before you break my heart. *Think it over.*

Who would have ever thought this classic tune by the Supremes could apply to so much more than a girlfriend warning her wayward beau? Contained within the melody is a very powerful statement: "Think it over."

I wonder how many bad choices and severe consequences could have been averted if that three-word statement had been applied.

Sometimes we can muster up the gumption to *think it over* on our own and redirect our steps away from the slippery slope of compromise. But, more times than not, we need measures of accountability.

For me, one of the most effective accountability measures has been mutually tracking progress with friends. I have one friend who started ahead of me and who has been an invaluable source of encouragement and perspective. She's the one I mentioned earlier, with the nutritionist.

---

ned across the table one day and said, "Lysa, if you do this healthy eating plan, it will work." I clung to that statement when I had a little breakdown.

The first three weeks of my new eating plan, things went well. I only struggled with being hungry the first ten days. At the start of week four, I think my body went through sugar withdrawals. I'm not kidding.

All my systems were out of whack. I felt like I had the flu one day, severe allergies the next, and then stomach issues for a week after that. It was definitely my angry little self, demanding I give my body some SUGAR NOW!

I felt awful. I could hardly exercise. I had to nap—and if you know me in real life, you know what a shocker that is! Part of me was ready to throw in the towel, head to the boxed-brownie aisle at the store, and ask if anyone knew how to hook up an IV line between me and Betty Crocker.

We must be aware that desperation breeds degradation. In other words, when what is lacking in life goes from annoyance to anxiety, we run the risk of compromising in ways we never thought we would.

I find it interesting that a verse many of us know and quote—how the devil prowls about like a roaring lion looking for someone to devour—is tucked right at the end of a passage that says, "Cast all your anxiety on him because he cares for you. Be self-controlled and alert" (1 Peter 5:7–8).

You see, when we determine to get healthy, we will

have to give up certain things and change our habits. Doing this can make us feel anxious. That's why we must have friends to help us remember that what we're giving up in the short term will help us get what we really want in the long term. If we forget to be self-controlled and alert, we are prime targets for Satan to usher us right away from the new standards we've set in our life. That's degradation.

Yes, desperation breeds degradation.

A person who thinks she would never steal gets into a financial bind and suddenly finds herself skimming money from the register at work.

A person who thinks she'd never have sex before marriage feels physically pressured by someone she desperately wants love from and suddenly finds herself in bed with him.

A person committed to getting healthy forgets to pack her healthy snacks and suddenly feels it's urgent to zip by the vending machine and grab a candy bar just this one time.

Be aware and be on guard, sweet sister. Know that these are schemes the devil has devised to lure you away from your commitments. Find a friend who can speak rationality into your irrational impulses. A friend who will hold you accountable, speak the truth in love, and pray for you.

Look at the great example of how desperation breeds degradation in the Old Testament story of Esau. Esau, the older of two twins, was a skillful hunter, while the younger twin, Jacob, was more of a homebody. The Scriptures say:

> Once when Jacob was cooking some stew, Esau came in from the open country, famished. He said to Jacob, "Quick, let me have some of that red stew! I'm famished!" (That is why he was also called Edom.)
>
> Jacob replied, "First sell me your birthright."
>
> "Look, I am about to die," Esau said. "What good is the birthright to me?"
>
> But Jacob said, "Swear to me first." So he swore an oath to him, selling his birthright to Jacob.
>
> Then Jacob gave Esau some bread and some lentil stew. He ate and drank, and then got up and left.
>
> So Esau despised his birthright. (Genesis 25:29–34)

The thing that strikes me about this story is how much Esau gave up for just a few moments of physical satisfaction. He sacrificed what was good in the long term for what felt good in the short term. He gave up who he was in a moment of desperation.

Had a true friend of Esau's heard this interaction with Jacob, surely he would have spoken some rationality into Esau's irrational impulses.

That's what my friend was for me—a voice of reason,

stability, and rationality. While she held fast with her assurances, I cried. Cried *tears*, y'all—big tears over the lack of sugar and salty treats and the temporary highs they always gave me. After calling her, I'd lie down on my bathroom floor and beg God for His help. To say I was miserable was an understatement. But if she could press through her withdrawal days, so could I.

Then the day after my worst day, all my symptoms vanished. Suddenly I felt great. My body was strong, my emotions were in check, my energy level was sky high. Just like my friend said would happen.

Amazing.

Persevering through my breakdown ushered me into a sweet place of breakthrough, and suddenly I started seeing tangible results. It felt so good not to dread getting dressed in the morning. It was a major perk to wear clothes that actually fit. Granted, they were still my "big clothes," but being able to put them on with comfort and ease was a great step in the right direction.

It also was crucial to have the accountability of another friend, Holly, who started this healthy eating plan at the same time I did. We both knew it would be hard, so we committed to praying for each other as well as holding each other accountable. Every day we talked about what we'd be eating. Then weekly we reported our weights to each other. We talked through each struggle, each temptation that seemed so consuming, each step both good and bad.

Knowing I couldn't hide little cheats here and there

from Holly kept me from slipping. I couldn't stand the thought of having to tell her I'd messed up—so I didn't. Our motto became, "If it's not part of our plan, we don't put it in our mouths."

If you don't have a friend who is willing to take this journey with you by changing her eating habits, don't be discouraged. Find a friend who is willing to take the journey with you in prayer. Be honest with her about your struggles and ask her to commit to praying fervently for you and with you.

Honestly, I *never, ever* thought I could really give up eating bread, pasta, rice, potatoes, and sugar. But seeing the success of friends ahead of me and knowing I had someone who was willing to sacrifice with me gave my brain permission to stop—in the name of love—and think it over.

While you'll have to find a friend to either do a healthy eating plan with you or one who will pray you through it, let me be that voice that reaches across your doubts to say, "If you follow the healthy eating plan you've chosen, it will work and it most certainly will be worth it." And when you get into possible trouble with temptation, remember to "stop in the name of love." Let your love for your friends who are standing with you and your love for the Lord, who wants you to honor Him in the way you treat your body, make you think it over.

So, are you ready? Take time to prayerfully consider the right healthy eating plan for you. Talk to your friends to see who might be willing to join you. And then start walking toward the healthy life that's possible for you.

05

made for more

When I was a senior in high school, I was invited to a sorority party by a friend who'd graduated the year before me.

Cool doesn't even begin to describe what I felt as my pink jelly shoes and I made our way into that party. By the end of the night, my friend and I were giggling over the attention given to us by two good-looking college boys. As the party died down, they invited us over to their place.

Part of me was so flattered, I wanted to go. A much bigger part of me didn't. But plans got made, and before I knew it we were getting into their car and driving away.

I was not a Christian at this point in my life. Not even close. And I certainly can't say I'd ever heard God speak to me, but in the midst of this situation, I did.

This isn't you, Lysa. You were made for more than this.

Truth. A gift of truth. Planted deep within me when God personally knit me together. Untied and presented at just the right time.

I wound up making an excuse for a quick exit and walked back to my car alone that night. I mentally beat lf up for acting like an immature high schooler who couldn't handle being a college party girl. But looking back, I want to stand up on a chair and clap, clap, clap for my high school self!

There were other seasons of my growing-up years when I heard this truth loud and clear within the confines of my soul and, sadly, I refused to listen. These were the darkest years of my life. I wasn't made to live a life that dishonors the Lord.

None of us are.

You were made for more, Lysa. You were made for more. I remembered it especially in those early weeks of my new healthy eating adventure when I was tempted by one million assaults on my sugar-deprived taste buds. I just kept mentally repeating . . . *made for more . . . made for more.*

What a great truth for us all. What a great truth to use while rewriting the "go-to" scripts that play in our heads every time we're tempted. Rewriting the go-to scripts is one of the most crucial steps toward permanent progress.

We have to rewrite the excuses, the rationalizations, the "I'll do better tomorrow" escape clauses by getting into the habit of saying other things. And the first of these is, "I was made for more." Wrapped in this truth is a wisdom and revelation that unlocks great power available to all Christians.

And isn't power what girls in pursuit of making healthy life changes really need? We need a power beyond our frail attempts and fragile resolve. A power greater than our taste buds, hormones, temptations, and our inborn female demand for chocolate.

Read what the apostle Paul wrote about this amazing power available to us, and note the emphasized phrases, which we'll take a closer look at in a moment:

> *I keep asking* that the God of our Lord Jesus Christ, the *glorious Father,* may give you the Spirit of wisdom and revelation, *so that you may know him better.* I pray that the eyes of your heart may be enlightened in order that you may know the hope to which he has called you, the riches of his glorious inheritance in his holy people, and *his incomparably great power for us* who believe. (Ephesians 1:17–19, emphasis added)

Now I realize it is hard to take a passage like this, hold it up to a decadent piece of chocolate cake, and instantly feel the power to walk away. But if we unpack this passage and then practice its truth, it's amazing how empowered we'll be. So, let's take a closer look at some key words and phrases.

Be Persistent: "I Keep Asking"

We must ask God to join us in this journey. And this won't be a one-time exercise. Paul asked over and over and over again for wisdom. So should we. We need to ask for God's wisdom, revelation, and intervening power to be an integral part of our food choices from now on.

Why not make this a daily prayer—first thing in the morning—before we've eaten a thing: "God, I recognize I am made for more than the vicious cycle of being ruled by food. I need to eat to live, not live to eat. So, I keep asking for Your wisdom to know what to eat and Your indwelling power to walk away from things that aren't beneficial for me."

Embrace a True Identity: "Glorious Father"

The phrase "glorious Father" indicates our relationship to God and answers the question, "*Why* are we made for more?" We are made for more because we are children of God. For years I identified myself not by my relationship with God but by my circumstances. I was . . .

Lysa, the *broken* girl from a broken home.

Lysa, the girl *rejected* by her father.

Lysa, the girl *sexually abused* by a grandfather figure.

Lysa, the girl who *walked away from God* after the death of her sister.

Lysa, the girl who *had an abortion* after a string of bad relationships.

Then one day I read a list of who God says ⸺ ....
What a stark contrast to the way I saw myself! I finally
realized I didn't have to be defined by my circumstances.
Instead, I could live in the reality of who my glorious
heavenly Father says I am:

Lysa, the *forgiven* child of God. (Romans 3:24)
Lysa, the *set-free* child of God. (Romans 8:1–2)
Lysa, the *accepted* child of God. (John 1:12)
Lysa, the *holy child* of God. (1 Corinthians 1:30)
Lysa, the *made-new* child of God. (2 Corinthians
5:17)
Lysa, the *loved* child of God. (Ephesians 1:4)
Lysa, the *confident* child of God. (Ephesians 3:12)
Lysa, the *victorious* child of God. (Romans 8:37)

I was made to be set free—holy, new, loved, and confident. Because of this, I can't allow myself to partake in
anything that negates my true identity. Be it a relationship in which someone makes me feel less than my true
identity or a vicious food cycle that leaves me defeated
and imprisoned, I must remember I was made for more.

Find the Deeper Reason: "So That You May Know Him Better"

Did you catch the real reason for embracing our true identity? It's not just so we can feel better about ourselves or to help us make healthier choices. It's not even to help us operate as victorious children of God. And it's certainly not so we can slip into smaller jeans and lose the muffin tops, although these are all wonderful benefits.

The real reason is "so that you may know Him better."

There is a deeper purpose behind our disciplined commitment. Making this connection—between being made for more and getting to know God better—helps this whole adventure be less about food and lifestyle choices and more about embracing a chance for deep, wonderful connections with God.

Discover a Hope and Power Like No Other: "That the Eyes of Your Heart May Be Enlightened"

Enlighten literally means "to shed light upon."[2] In other words, the apostle Paul asked that light be shed upon our hearts so we can more clearly recognize the hope and power available to us.

We are made for the same hope and power that raised Christ from the dead. We've covered Ephesians 1:17–19, but we must look at what follows: "That power is the same as the mighty strength he exerted when he raised Christ from the dead and seated him at his right hand in the heavenly realms" (vv. 19–20). This is the power available to us! The same power that raised Jesus from the dead! It may not feel like we have this power, but we do—*you* do. And I pray that each time you proclaim, "I am made for more," all the power-packed truths within that statement rush into your heart.

We were made for more than excuses and vicious cycles. We can taste success. Experience truth. Choose to stay on the path of perseverance. Build one success on top of another. And our eating habits can be totally transformed as we operate in the hope and power that's like no other.

growing closer to God

I was once at a conference doing a question-and-answer session when someone asked, "How do you grow close to God?"

Great question. Possible answers swirled about in my mind. I ultimately answered, "By making the choice to deny ourselves something that is permissible but not beneficial. And making this intentional sacrifice for the sole purpose of growing closer to God. After all, Jesus Himself said, 'If anyone wants to come after Me, he must deny himself, take up his cross daily, and follow Me'" (Luke 9:23 NASB).

By way of example, I shared how I was intentionally sacrificing sugar and processed things that, once consumed, turn into sugar in my body. Yes, I was doing it to get healthy. But the deeper reason for choosing to purify myself was to help me grow closer to God.

My answer was real, vulnerable, and honest. Maybe a little too honest. The women in the audience gasped when I said I was in a season of sacrificing sugar. It wasn't two seconds later that a conference attendee grabbed the audience microphone and blurted out, "Well, if Jesus called Himself the Bread of Life, I can't see how sugar and processed carbs are bad at all!"

The audience erupted with laughter.

I forced a smile, but I felt smaller than a wart on the end of an ant's nose.

They didn't get it.

Or maybe I didn't get it. Was I just a foolish, Jesus-chasing girl who mistakenly believed my desires to please Him with this food battle would somehow help me grow closer to Him?

Yes, I want to lose weight. But this journey really is about learning to tell myself no and make wiser choices daily. And somehow becoming a woman of self-discipline honors God and helps me live the godly characteristic of self-control, which is among the fruit of the Spirit (the evidence of God's Spirit being in you) listed in Galatians 5:22–23. In the end, pursuing self-control does help my heart feel purer and closer to Jesus to receive what He wants for me each day . . . instead of clogged with guilty feelings about my poor choices.

But self-control is hard. We don't like to deny ourselves. We don't think it's necessary. We make excuses and declare, "That's nice for you, but I could never give that up." And if we're relying on ourselves, that's true. But there's another level to self-control that too few of us find.

Before the apostle Paul listed the fruit of the Spirit in his letter to the churches in Galatia, he described a power to us that goes way beyond self-control: "So I ~~say,~~ *by the Spirit*, and you will not gratify the desires of the sinful nature" (Galatians 5:16, emphasis added). In other words, live with the willingness to walk away when the Holy Spirit nudges you and says, "That food choice is permissible but not beneficial—so don't eat it."

Not *sinful*—please hear me on this. Food isn't sinful. But when food is what Satan holds up in front us and says, "You'll never be free from this battle. You aren't capable of self-control with food," we must see that its inappropriate consumption can be his lure to draw our hearts into a place of defeat. For others it will be sex outside marriage, the inappropriate consumption of alcohol, illegal drugs, or some other physical means.

The obvious question, then, is how can we tune in to these nudges of the Holy Spirit? How can we "live by the Spirit"?

First, we have to know where the Spirit is and what He gives us. If we know Jesus as our personal Savior, the Bible teaches that we have the Holy Spirit living in us (Romans 8:11), infusing our lives with power that is beyond what we could muster up on our own.

Now then, how do we live by this Spirit and heed His voice of wisdom and caution? Here's what the apostle Paul said: "Let us keep in step with the Spirit" (Galatians 5:25). In other words, we read the Bible with the intention of practicing what we read while asking the Holy Spirit to direct us in knowing how to do this.

I often pray this prayer: "I need wisdom to make wise choices. I need insight to remember the words I've read in Scripture. I need power beyond what I can find on my own." It's not a magic prayer. I still have to make the choice to walk away from the source of my temptation.

And making that choice is sometimes really hard; I won't deny that.

Like when I'm in line at Starbucks. The barista takes my coffee order and then waves her hand like an enticing wand, directing my attention to a case full of delights that make a girl's taste buds dance. Seriously dance. Like the rumba, tango, and a snappy little quick step all in a row. My taste buds dance around while begging like a small child in the candy aisle.

"Would you like something to go with your coffee?" she asks.

Of course I'd like something—I'd like two or three somethings! And I'll be completely honest, it's in moments like these that I want to ask Eve to clarify one simple thing. Please tell me that something got lost in translation and what was really dangling from that tree limb all those years ago were treats like this. I'm just saying.

Anyhow. Like I said, it's not easy. It's not easy relying on the Holy Spirit to direct us into wise choices. It's not easy to dare to actually live a life in which we put Scripture in action. Especially scriptures about self-control.

It's not easy but it *is* possible.

We serve a compassionate God. A God who knew

food would be a major stumbling block in our all-out pursuit of Him. So He's given us great gifts in the Holy Spirit, Jesus, and the Bible to help us.

Let's look at two specific aspects of faith that God warns us must not be allowed to be eclipsed by food: our calling and our commitment.

Our Calling

Whenever we feel defeated by an issue, it can make us feel unable to follow God completely. Sometimes this would haunt me and make me feel insecure in my ministry to women. Have you ever felt this way in your struggle with food? I bet you never dreamed the story of the Samaritan woman might provide some very sweet encouragement.

Right smack dab in the middle of one of the longest recorded interactions Jesus had with a woman, He started talking about food. Food! And I'd never picked up on it before. Somehow, in all my exposure to her story over the years, I missed Jesus' crucial teaching that spiritual nourishment is even more important than physical nourishment. He said, "My food . . . is to do the will of him who sent me and to finish his work" (John 4:34). And then He said, "I tell you, open your eyes and look at the fields! They are ripe for harvest" (v. 35).

There is a bigger plan here! Don't get distracted by physical food. Don't think physical food can satisfy the

longing of your soul. Only Jesus can do that. Our
were created to crave Him and love others to Him. See,
there are many people waiting to hear the message of your
calling. Don't get stuck in defeat and held back from it.

Food can fill our stomachs but never our souls.

Possessions can fill our houses but never our hearts.

Sex can fill our nights but never our hunger for love.

Children can fill our days but never our identities.

Only by being filled with authentic soul food from
Jesus—following Him and telling others about Him—
will our souls ever be truly satisfied. And breaking free
from consuming thoughts about food allows us to see and
pursue our calling with more confidence and clarity.

Our Commitment

I love God. I've loved God for a long time. But it took God
quite a while to get my attention with my food issues. One
of the things He used to get my attention is pointing out
things in the Bible I'd never really noticed before.

Philippians is often called the book of joy. This sec-
tion of Scripture starts off easy enough:

> One thing I do: Forgetting what is behind and
> straining toward what is ahead, I press on toward
> the goal to win the prize for which God has
> called me heavenward in Christ Jesus.

All of us, then, who are mature should take such a view of things. And if on some point you think differently, that too God will make clear to you. Only let us live up to what we have already attained. (3:13–16)

Love those verses. I want to forget what is behind! I want to press on toward the goal! I want to win the prize! I want to be mature! So we clap our hands at the end of that message and promise to do some prize-winning pressing on for Jesus.

But wait. Don't file out of class just yet. If we look just a tad further in this chapter, we'll find a telling verse about food:

For, as I have often told you before and now tell you again even with tears, many live as enemies of the cross of Christ. Their destiny is destruction, their god is their stomach, and their glory is in their shame. Their mind is on earthly things. (vv. 18–19)

Oh dear. Those are some stinging, toe-stubbing words. Words that don't exactly make us want to stand up and clap. But they are there and we must pay attention.

When the apostle Paul said, "Their god is their stomach," he meant that food can become so consuming that people find themselves ruled by it. To make that

38

practical, if we find that certain foods are impo
walk away from—we can't or won't deny ourse..es an
unhealthy choice—then it's a clue we are being ruled by
this food on some level. Being ruled by something other
than God diminishes our commitment and will make us
feel increasingly distant from Him.

Being ruled by anything other than God is something God takes quite seriously. And so should I. I
don't want to live as an enemy of the cross of Christ.
I don't want to live resistant to the power Christ's death
and resurrection provides just because I can't walk away
from my unhealthy cravings.

Thankfully, Paul's words to the Philippians don't end
in verse 19. There's good news:

> But our citizenship is in heaven. And we eagerly
> await a Savior from there, the Lord Jesus Christ,
> who, by the power that enables him to bring
> everything under his control, will transform our
> lowly bodies so that they will be like his glorious
> body (vv. 20–21)

Now I can clap again. I want His power to help me
bring everything—*everything*—under His control. I want
my lowly body to be transformed. I want to be in the process of becoming more and more like Jesus. It reestablishes
that God, not food, is in control of me. That helps keep
me undivided in my commitment to Him.

So, is this eating-healthier journey really something that can help us grow closer to God?

Yes, I believe it is. I stand by the answer I gave at the conference that day. And while making the intentional choice to deny myself unhealthy food options probably isn't the most popular route to growing closer to God, it is a route nonetheless. A thrilling, hard, practical, courageous, satisfying spiritual journey with great physical benefits.

not defined by
the numbers

A few years ago, I was in an exercise class when the gal next to me leaned over and started to tell me that she'd spent the weekend with her sister. They'd had a good time, but she came away concerned. It seems this sister had gained quite a bit of weight. I was half listening and half straining to crunch my screaming stomach. Suddenly I snapped to attention when she quipped, "I mean I can hardly believe it. I think my sister now weighs like 150 pounds."

I didn't know whether to laugh out loud or just keep my hilarious little secret to myself. The scandalous weight that horrified my workout friend was the exact number that had greeted me that very morning on my scale.

About this time, the exercise instructor directed us to grab our jump ropes, which abruptly ended the conversation. But for the rest of class, I couldn't wipe the smile off my face. In that moment I had a small victory over an identity disorder I'd battled for a very long time.

Like many women, I'd struggled with a flawed perception of myself. My sense of identity and worth were dependent on the wrong things—my circumstances or my weight or whether I yelled at the kids that day or what other people thought of me. If I sensed I wasn't measuring up, I kicked into either withdrawal mode or fix-it mode. Withdrawal mode made me pull back from relationships, fearing others' judgments. I built walls around my heart to keep people at a distance. Fix-it mode made me over-analyze other people's every word and expression, looking for ways to manipulate their opinions to be more favorable toward me.

Both of these are crazy modes to be in.

I found great joy in realizing that my workout buddy's statement hadn't rattled me. I wasn't at my goal weight, but I was in the process of investing wisely in my health and spiritual growth. I had been diligently filling my heart and mind with God's truths, and these truths were protecting me. In this moment, I could feel the Holy Spirit filling me with a calm reassurance. And it felt absolutely great to say to myself, "One hundred and fifty pounds isn't where I want to be, but it's better than where I started. It's tangible evidence of progress—and progress is good!"

I got a faint remembrance of some verses I'd recently marked in my Bible. Later I looked them up, and though God was clearly talking to a ruler who probably had very different struggles than I do, I found the words amazingly comforting. Here is what I heard God saying to me through the words He spoke to Isaiah:

"I will go before you" . . . *I [God] knew this comment would be made in exercise class this morning.*

"and will level the mountains" . . . *and that's why the Holy Spirit prompted you to remember these verses: to protect you from what could have been a huge hurt to your heart.*

"I will break down gates of bronze and cut through bars of iron" . . . *I will break through the lies that could have imprisoned you and made you doubt your true worth.*

"I will give you hidden treasures, riches stored in secret places" . . . *In the most unlikely places I will bless your efforts and reward your perseverance with indications of your victory.*

"so that you may know that I am the LORD, the God of Israel, who summons you by name" . . . *I love you, Lysa. I loved you when you weighed almost 200 pounds. I loved you at 167. I love you at 150. And no number on the scale will ever change that. I'm not taking you on this journey because I need you to weigh less but because I desire for you to be healthy in every sense of the word. I know your name, Lysa. Now rest in the security of My name and all that it means to your identity.* (Isaiah 45:2–3, italicized words added) you see why it's so important to fill our hearts and minds with God's words? How vital it is to make His truth the foundation not only for our identity but for how we deal with food? The Holy Spirit uses God's words stored up inside us to nudge us, remind us, redirect us, empower us, and lead us on to victory.

I wish I could give you a more definitive formula. Something a little more packaged and step-by-step and not so reliant on having to make a choice to listen to the Holy Spirit. But one thing I can assure you: God wants to be in communication with us. And, if you dedicate this journey to God, He promises the Holy Spirit will be with you every step of the way. That means you have access to a power beyond your own.

So because of God's truth, this Jesus-loving girl wasn't defeated by my workout friend's remark. I didn't melt into a puddle of tears. This conversation about a 150-pound sister didn't define me in any way. I simply chuckled and moved on while humming that song from the animated movie *Shark Tale*, "I Like Big Butts and I Cannot Lie." It was truly a glorious life moment for me. This interaction was living proof I was finally on a healing path.

Here's another step for growing closer to God that we cannot miss: we grow closer to God as we learn to look and act more and more like Him. The Bible calls this participating in His divine nature.

Not only do our actions need to reflect the self-control the Holy Spirit affords us, but our sense of identity

needs to reflect His presence in our lives. Here's h
apostle Peter presented this truth:

> His divine power has given us everything we
> need for a godly life through our knowledge of
> him who called us by his own glory and good-
> ness. Through these he has given us his very
> great and precious promises, so that through
> them you may participate in the divine nature,
> having escaped the corruption in the world
> caused by evil desires.
>
> For this very reason, make every effort to
> add to your faith goodness; and to goodness,
> knowledge; and to knowledge, self-control;
> and to self-control, perseverance; and to per-
> severance, godliness; and to godliness, mutual
> affection; and to mutual affection, love. For if
> you possess these qualities in increasing mea-
> sure, they will keep you from being ineffective
> and unproductive in your knowledge of our
> Lord Jesus Christ. (2 Peter 1:3–8)

That's a lot of text, so let me summarize the principles
in these verses that relate to our struggles with food and
identity:

- God's divine power has given us everything we
  need to experience victory in our struggles.

- We are to reflect a divine nature—a secure identity in Christ—which helps us escape the corruption of the world and avoid evil desires.
- It is through biblical promises that we find the courage to deny unhealthy desires.
- Getting healthy is not just about having faith, goodness, and knowledge. We have to add to that foundation by choosing to be self-controlled and choosing to persevere even when the journey gets really hard.
- These qualities keep us from being ineffective and unproductive in our pursuit of healthy eating and, even more importantly, in our pursuit of growing closer to God.
- If we make the choice to be Jesus girls who offer our willingness to exercise self-control and perseverance to the glory of God, we can lose weight, get healthy, and walk in confidence that it is possible to escape the cycle of losing and gaining back again. We can be victorious. We can step on the scale and accept the numbers for what they are—an indication of how much our bodies weigh—and not an indication of our worth.

May I just repeat that last little line? *I am a Jesus girl who can step on the scale and see the numbers as an indication of how much my body weighs and not as an indication of my worth.*

Sister, if you are like me, you have places where parents, peers, friends, and foes have purposely or inadvertently hurt you with their comments. And sometimes those comments rattle around in your heart and mind and chip away at your worth.

That day in the gym, I could have let the words "I can hardly believe it. She must weigh like 150 pounds" bump around and cause great damage. Instead, I took that comment and held it up to the truths the Holy Spirit was whispering. Like the apostle Peter said, we have been given everything we need for life and godliness. My classmate's inadvertent statement was not life and it was not godly. Therefore, I didn't have to internalize it. I could leave it on the gym floor and walk away.

That statement didn't belong to me. That statement wasn't my issue. I had a choice to make. I could feed that comment and let it grow into an identity crusher, or I could see it for what it was, a careless comment. Just like I can make the choice to leave the cookies in the bakery case and the chips on the grocery store shelf, I could make the choice to walk away from that remark. That's what the apostle Paul was talking about when he said, "We demolish arguments and every pretension that sets itself up against the knowledge of God, and we take captive every thought to make it obedient to Christ" (2 Corinthians 10:5).

We can literally say to any comment or thought, "Are you true? Are you beneficial? Are you necessary?" And if the answer is no, then we don't open the doors of our hearts.

I love these verses. I love these truths. I love my identity as a Jesus girl. And I love not being defined by numbers.

0 8

making peace with the realities of my body

I have a high school memory that haunted me for years. There was a boy with whom I was completely smitten. When the lights dimmed at school dances, somewhere between "My Sharona" and "Walk Like an Egyptian," inevitably came the sounds of Hall and Oates's "Your Kiss Is on My List." I had a list and he was at the very top.

The only problem was that my crush had a list of his own and I hadn't even made the cut. To him, we were just friends. Put that little combo together and it was a formula for heartbreak.

Then came the moment that more than twenty years later, I can still recall as if it happened yesterday. List Boy comes and sits beside me at the school dance. I try to play cool and act like I'm surprised to see him. Like I hadn't noticed him all night, though I had secretly kept an eye on his every move since he'd walked in. We exchange chit-chat for a few minutes.

We are only speaking very simple words, but inside

---

of me a whole different thing is happening. My heart is beating out of my chest; my mind is leaping through pages of our future together—our first dance, our engagement, our wedding. Right as I'm getting around to naming our first three children, he drops a bomb on me.

He says he thinks I'm pretty cute, but it's too bad I have big ankles, otherwise we might be able to go out sometime.

"Excuse me? Did you just say I have big beautiful eyes? Surely you didn't just say *ankles?*"

"No," he replies, "I actually said TANKLES."

Seriously . . . TANKLES! I could have imagined him never asking me out because of my frizzy hair or my zits or my braces . . . *all of that would eventually change.* But my ankles? Well, they would be my constant companion for life.

I eventually matured past my ankles bothering me every minute of every day. Just about the time when they were merely a *weekly* point of contention, I decided to have a little conversation with God about my ankles. I told Him this was a silly thing to bring up, but I really needed to have a better perspective on the whole tankle ankle situation.

I think the Lord had actually been eager for me to discuss this with Him. He was quick to answer my question with a question.

God: "Are you clumsy, Lysa?"
Lysa: "Yes, Lord. I am very clumsy."
God: "Have you ever twisted your ankle?"

50

Lysa: "Never."

God: "Wouldn't it bug you to constantly twist your ankle and be put out of commission?"

Lysa: "Yes, very much."

God: "Lysa, I have perfectly equipped you with ankles of strength and convenience. Be thankful."

The conversation wasn't as clear-cut and back and forth as that. And no, I didn't audibly hear God's voice. But this is the message I got as I sat quietly and prayed about this. Maybe you could try having a similar "quiet time" with God about whatever your tankle equivalent is and see what He reveals to you.

I don't know a woman alive who is completely happy with her body. Not me. Probably not you. And not my friend Karen Ehman, who lost more than one hundred pounds.

Karen is one of my most favorite people to dialogue with about weight loss. Karen grew up with a single mom who truly loved her but couldn't always be as available as she wanted to be for her daughter. Many days she'd try to fill the gap of her absence by telling Karen she'd left a box of treats on the counter as she rushed off to work another shift.

Treats became Karen's comfort—what she'd turn to when she was lonely, sad, or stressed. This pattern became deeply ingrained in Karen, and as the years went by, she ended up in what felt like an impossibly obese state. Through a series of medical scares and reality checks, Karen joined Weight Watchers and lost one hundred pounds. And for three years, she was able to stick with it and keep the weight off.

Then her husband lost his job. They had to sell their home. Other stresses mounted, and everything started spinning out of control. Suddenly her old patterns of comfort seemed appealing again. Plus, being at her goal weight and still having to watch what she ate without the reward of watching the scale numbers go down wasn't as fun. What started as one treat turned into many. Five extra pounds turned into thirty, and Karen felt the old pangs of defeat tempting her to make a complete reversal of all her progress.

It was time to get serious again, but boy was it hard the second time around! She knew some things would have to be different. The biggest was shifting her motivation from the delight of seeing the diminishing numbers on the scale to the delight of obedience to God.

On one of her "Weight Loss Wednesday" blog posts, she wrote something I found incredibly insightful and profound:

> I was very hopeful as I hopped on the scale this morning. I kept track of my food, exercised five days at the gym for 30–45 minutes, and my jeans were zipping up much easier than expected. So,

I whipped the scale out of its locked-down location (hopping on the scale more than once a week proves often to be detrimental to me) and it said . . .

I lost 1.8 pounds.

A measly 1.8 pounds! What!?! I was sure it would say at least two or maybe even three. I felt gypped. And I felt like running to the kitchen to make a frozen waffle or two so I could slather it with real butter, spread it with some Peter Pan, and douse it with a load of pure maple syrup to drown my sorrows.

Then I stopped and remembered what I felt the Lord saying this week.

Define your week by obedience, not by a number on the scale. . . .

So, I had to stop and ask myself the following questions:

- Did I overeat this week on any day? No.
- Did I move more and exercise regularly? Yes. . . .
- Did I eat in secret or out of anger or frustration? No.
- Did I feel that, at any time, I ran to food instead of to God? Nope.
- *Before* I hopped on the scale, did I think I'd had a successful, God-pleasing week? Yep!

So, why oh why do I get so tied up in a stupid number? And why did I almost let it trip me up and send me to the kitchen for a 750-calorie binge? . . .

Sweet friends, we need to define ourselves by our obedience, not a number on the scale.

Okay?

Pinky promise?

Good.

We are all in this thing together.

And we *will* get the weight off, even if it is 1.8 pounds at a time![3]

I love the questions Karen tackled. What a great list of questions for me to ask when, though I'm at my goal weight, it's still necessary for me to wear Spanx with some of my dress pants. Or when my tankles remind me skirts aren't my best wardrobe option.

The body God has given me is good. It's not perfect, nor will it ever be. I still have cellulite. I still have tankles. And though I eat healthy, there are no guarantees—I'm just as susceptible as the next gal to cancer or some other disease. But my body is a gift. A good gift for which I am thankful. Being faithful in taking care of this gift by walking according to God's plans gives me renewed strength to keep a healthy view of my body. And so, like the psalmist, I can pray this prayer of thanksgiving for the body I have and mean it:

Praise the LORD, my soul;
> all my inmost being, praise his
> > holy name.
Praise the LORD, O my soul,
> and forget not all his benefits—
who forgives all your sins
> and heals all your diseases,
who redeems your life from the pit
> and crowns you with love and
> > compassion,
who satisfies your desires with good
> things
> > so that your youth is renewed
> > > like the eagle's.

> > > > (Psalm 103:1–5)

It's so easy to get laser focused on what we see as wrong with our bodies. I knew I could eat healthy and exercise the rest of my life and still have tankles. In the grand scheme of things, this is a shallow concern. But, if I allowed my brain to park in a place of dissatisfaction about any part of my body, it would give Satan just enough room to move in with his lie that strips me of motivation: *Your body is never going to look the way you want it to look, so why sacrifice so much? Your discipline is in vain.* That's why I have to seek the Lord's perspective and, as Psalm 103 reminds us, "forget not all his benefits."

When I studied this scripture and decided to rest in the reality of what a good gift my body is, for the first time in my life I thanked God for making me just the way He made me. I am able to look at airbrushed, skinny-ankled women on TV or in the magazines and be happy for them without loathing myself.

I've found my beautiful. And I like my beautiful. I don't have to hold my beautiful up to others and view it with a critical eye. As Ralph Waldo Emerson once said, "Though we travel the world over to find the beautiful, we must carry it with us or we find it not."[4]

but exercise makes me want to cry

Can I just be honest? Exercise, especially cardio, has always been such a battle for me. I would halfheartedly do something physical a couple of times a week, hating every minute of it. The most frustrating part was, halfhearted efforts only produced mediocre results. Over the years, I started slipping further and further away from an active lifestyle.

Eventually I wondered whether I should just resign myself to being out of shape. I wondered, *Have I reached an age and stage of life where losing weight and getting fit are impossible?*

The many extra pounds that had crept onto my body could easily be justified. After all, I'd birthed three children. (I even seemed to gain weight with the two we adopted.) This was my season of raising kids, not lifting weights. I was too busy running carpools to run for exercise. But, in the quiet of my heart, I wasn't settled. I didn't feel good physically or emotionally. I would catch

---

myself standing in front of the bathroom mirror in tears many mornings, lamenting over which pants could best hide my bulge. I cried out to God and admitted it was crazy to get emotional about my pants, for heaven's sake. I wanted to rise above this vain issue and be comfortable with who I was.

The tide of justifications would roll back in, only this time with a spiritual twist: *The world has sold us women a bill of goods that to be good we have to be skinny. I am too concerned with my spiritual growth to be distracted by petty issues such as weight and exercise. God loves me just the way I am.*

While the spiritual justifications also sounded good, if I was honest with myself, my issue was plain and simple: a lack of self-control. I could sugarcoat it and justify it all day long, but the truth was, I didn't have a weight problem; I had a spiritual problem. I depended on food for comfort more than I depended on God. And I was simply too lazy to make time to exercise.

Ouch. That truth hurt.

So the day after Mother's Day a couple of years ago, I got up first thing in the morning and went running. Well, the word *running* should be used very loosely for what I actually did. I got out and moved my body quicker than I had in a long time. And you know what? I hated it. Exercise just made me want to cry.

It made me hot and sticky. It made my legs hurt and my lungs burn. Nothing about it was fun until after I

finished. But the feeling of accomplishment I felt after-
ward was fantastic! So, each day I would fight through the
tears and excuses and make the effort to run.

At first I could only slowly jog from one mailbox to
another—in a neighborhood where the houses are close
together, thank you very much. Every day I asked God
to give me the strength to stick with it this time. Slowly I
started to see little evidences of progress.

One day I went out for my version of a run and a
clear command from God rumbled in my heart: *Run until
you can't take another step. Do it not in your strength but in
Mine. Every time you want to stop, pray for that struggling
friend you just challenged not to give up, and take your own
advice—don't stop until I tell you to.*

I had a record up to that point of running three miles,
which I thought was quite stellar. But as I reached that
point in my run, my heart betrayed my aching body and
said, *Keep going.*

Each step thereafter, I had to pray and rely on God.
The more I focused on running toward God, the less I
thought about my desire to stop. And this verse from the
Psalms came to life:

> My flesh and my heart may fail,
>> but God is the strength of my
>> heart
> and my portion forever.

(73:26)

As I ran that day, I connected with God on a different level. I experienced what it meant to absolutely require God's faith to see something through. How many times have I claimed to be a woman of faith but rarely lived a life requiring faith? That day God didn't have me stop until I ran 8.6 miles.

Hear me out here. It was *my* legs that took every step. It was *my* energy being used. It was *my* effort that took me from 1 mile to 3 to 5 to 8.6. But it was *God's strength* replacing my excuses step by step by step.

For a mailbox-to-mailbox, crying-when-she-thought-of-exercising kind of girl, it was a modern-day miracle. I broke through the "I can't" barrier and expanded the horizons of my reality. Was it hard? Yes. Was it tempting to quit? Absolutely. Could I do this in my own strength? Never. But this really wasn't about running. It was about realizing the power of God taking over my complete weakness.

I should also note that I went back to my standard 3-mile track the next time I ran. But slowly I increased my daily runs to 4 miles and am very happy with that distance. Running 8.6 miles on a daily basis isn't realistic for me. But that one day, it was glorious. Especially because of what I discovered when I got home.

Since I'd been thinking of a verse from Psalms during my run, I grabbed my Bible as soon as I got home and opened it up to Psalm 86, in honor of my 8.6 miles. Here is part of what I read:

> Teach me your way, LORD,
>   and I will walk in your truth;
> give me an undivided heart,
>   that I may fear your name.
> I will praise you, LORD my God,
>   with all my heart;
>   I will glorify your name forever.

(vv. 11–12)

An undivided heart. That's what my whole journey in conquering my cravings was about.

When it comes to my body, I can't live with divided loyalties. I can either be loyal to honoring the Lord with my body or loyal to my cravings, desires, and many excuses for not exercising. The apostle Paul taught the Corinthians about this when he wrote: "Do you not know that your bodies are temples of the Holy Spirit, who is in you, whom you have received from God? You are not your own; you were bought at a price. Therefore honor God with your bodies" (1 Corinthians 6:19–20).

I found the most interesting story in the Old Testament about how serious God is about people taking care of the temples entrusted to them. Before the Holy Spirit was given to us and our bodies became the temples for God's presence, God was present with His people in a house of worship called a temple. The book of Haggai describes how one of the first things God's people did when they returned from exile in Babylon was to rebuild the temple.

They started with great enthusiasm and wonderful intentions but slowly slipped back into complacency and eventually stopped their work on the temple completely. Other things seemed more urgent, more appealing. Here's how God responded:

> This is what the LORD Almighty says: "These people say, 'The time has not yet come to rebuild the LORD's house.'"
>
> Then the word of the LORD came through the prophet Haggai: "Is it a time for you yourselves to be living in your paneled houses, while this house remains a ruin?"
>
> Now this is what the LORD Almighty says: "Give careful thought to your ways. You have planted much, but harvested little. You eat, but never have enough. You drink, but never have your fill. You put on clothes, but are not warm. You earn wages, only to put them in a purse with holes in it."
>
> This is what the LORD Almighty says: "Give careful thought to your ways. Go up into the mountains and bring down timber and build my house, so that I may take pleasure in it and be honored," says the LORD. (Haggai 1:2–8)

Oh, this reminds me just how divided my heart can be when it comes to taking care of my body, God's temple.

Just like these people, I could so easily say, "I'm not in a season where it's feasible to take care of my body. I just can't find the time between the kids, my work responsibilities, running a home, paying the bills, and all the day-to-day activities." But the Lord's strong caution is to "give careful thought to [our] ways" and to make time to "build [his] house" so that He may be honored.

God's people neglected building the temple for ten years. Each year something else seemed to be more important. For years, I did the same thing with exercise. Something else was always a higher priority.

However, if I were really honest, I'd have to admit I made time for what I wanted to make time for. I always seemed to find time to watch a favorite TV show or chat with a friend on the phone. Just the same, the Jews who returned from Babylon obviously had time to do things they really wanted to do while ignoring the home of the Lord.

There were consequences of failing to care for the Lord's temple: "Therefore, because of you the heavens have withheld their dew and the earth its crops" (v. 10). Now, I'm not saying God will cause bad things to happen to us if we don't exercise, but there are natural consequences for not taking care of our bodies. Be it more weight and less energy now or heart disease later, our choices matter in the physical and spiritual sense.

Spiritually, when I'm not taking care of my body, I feel much more weighed down by my stress and problems.

I have less energy to serve God and more challenging emotions to wade through when processing life.

I'm actually thankful now for a body and a metabolism that require me to exercise. I've given careful thought to my ways and determined that taking care of my temple is a top priority. I schedule it. I've learned to embrace the benefits instead of resisting the hardship. And though I never thought I'd say this, I love the feeling of accomplishment running gives me each day. Even if everything else in my day falls apart, I can smile and say, "Yes, but with the Lord's help, I ran four miles this morning!"

Running may not be your thing. So, find what is. My mom loves to say the best kind of exercise is the kind you'll do. I agree. And while I fully realize my temple may not be God's grandest dwelling, I want to lift up to the Lord whatever willingness I have each day and dedicate my exercise as a gift to Him and a gift to myself. This one act unifies my divided heart and reminds me of the deeper purposes for moving my body.

It's amazing how love can motivate us—especially when it's God's unreserved love matched with our undivided hearts.

10

this isn't fair!

A huge piece of bakery deliciousness sat in front of me. It was a combination of three desserts in one. One layer was cheesecake, one layer was ice cream cake, and in between those was a layer of brownie-like chocolate cake . . . all drizzled with some kind of fudge icing that was calling my name.

This was served to me while on a family vacation. At the time, I was at the beginning of my no-sugar adventure. I'd been doing great at home, but I'd been dropped into a place that was teeming with bakery things my mind could not even conceive of, while everyone around me could eat a pound of sugar a day and still look fit and trim.

I didn't want my family to miss out, so I told them to please enjoy. "I'm fine," I said with a carefree smile. But inside a totally different dialogue was playing in my mind: *It's not fair!*

I think this is one of the biggest tricks Satan plays on us girls to get us to give in to temptation.

Saying "it's not fair" has caused many a girl to toss aside what she knows is right for the temporary thrill of whatever it is that does seem fair. But the next day the sun will rise. As each band of light becomes brighter and brighter, the realization of the choice she made the night before becomes clearer and clearer.

Guilt floods her body.

Questions fill her mind.

Self-doubt wrecks her confidence.

And then comes the anger. Anger at herself. Anger at the object of her desire. Anger even at a mighty God who surely could have prevented this.

It's not fair that others can have this, do this, act this way.

It's not fair that God won't let us eat of the fruit of the tree in the middle of the garden . . . one little bite wouldn't be so bad, right?

It's not fair I can't buy that new thing I want. Just a little debt wouldn't be so bad, right?

It's not fair I have this body that requires I watch everything I eat when that girl eats junk and stays a size 4. One piece of cheesecake wouldn't be so bad, right?

It's not fair that we can't have sex before we're married when we're so in love. Experimenting one time wouldn't be so bad, right?

Our flesh buys right into Satan's lie that it's not fair for things to be withheld from us. So we bite into the forbidden fruit and allow Satan to write shame across our heart.

And whether we are talking about having premarital

sex or cheating on our diet, once we taste the forbidden fruit, we will crave it more than we craved it before—thereby giving temptation more and more power. And given enough power, temptation will consume our thoughts, redirect our actions, and demand our worship. Temptation doesn't take kindly to being starved.

I don't know what tempts you today. But I do know this vicious cycle, and I'm here to give you hope that it's possible to conquer it.

Just typing that sentence gives me chills. A few years ago, I wondered if it might ever be possible for me.

As I've mentioned, the eating plan I chose was a no-sugar, healthy-carbs-and-protein plan. Which doesn't sound so bad until you realize sugar is in just about everything we enjoy eating. Breads, pasta, potatoes, rice, not to mention all things bakery-licious.

So, sitting at that special dinner during my special vacation, I started to have a little pity party, and those words *It's not fair* crept into my brain.

In that instant I squirmed in my chair and thought, *I'll take just one little bite . . . maybe two . . . I've been so good . . . I even exercised this morning . . . this is vacation . . . everyone else is indulging . . . oh my stars, what are you doing, Lysa?!*

The sugar was like a siren of mythical tales, luring the ships over to rocky coves that would inevitably dash and destroy them. The seduction was smooth and seemingly innocent. But in that moment of temptation, I realized having a pity party was a clue I was relying on my own strength.

I had to grab hold of God's strength, and the only way to do that was to invite His power into this situation. In this case, I gave God control of the situation by mentally reciting, *I am made for more. I am made for more.*

I recalled pieces of scriptures I've tied to this go-to script and banked up in my heart. "I'm more than a conqueror." "With God all things are possible." "Let the peace of God reign in your heart." "Lead us not into temptation but *deliver* us from the evil one . . . "

The problem is, Satan hit me with a twist that left me momentarily shaky: *But this is a special time, Lysa. And special times deserve an exception to your normal parameters. It's not fair that you have to sacrifice. Look around you. No one else is sacrificing right now.*

It's at this exact point when the dieter on vacation indulges. The virgin sleeps with her prom date. The girl on a debt reduction plan pulls her credit card back out for a big sale. The alcoholic skips AA and heads off to the bar for her friend's fortieth birthday.

I needed a go-to script for this situation. So I lowered my head and prayed, "God, I am at the end of my strength here. The Bible says Your power is made perfect in weakness. This would be a really good time for that truth to be my reality. Help me see something else besides this temptation looming so large in front of me."

Suddenly a memory flashed across the screen of my

mind. I was sitting on my back deck with my teen son and his girlfriend at the time, having a deeply honest and gut-wrenching conversation. They had gotten into a bad situation and allowed things to go too far physically. While not every boundary line was crossed, they had crossed enough to scare them both. My advice to them was to think beyond the moment. Say out loud, "This feels good now, but how will I feel about this in the morning?"

That was it. I was challenged by the words and expectations I had placed on my son while not realizing how this same advice could be so powerful if applied to my area of struggle. I had my next go-to script, and as I recited it, God's power filled in the gap of my weakness.

Soon it was time to get up from the dinner table. I pushed back my chair, left the dessert untouched, and walked back to the room. And I've never felt so empowered in my life. Later, I looked up that verse about God's strength being a perfect match for my weakness:

> But [Jesus] said to me, "My grace is sufficient for you, for my power is made perfect in weakness." Therefore I will boast all the more gladly about my weaknesses, so that Christ's power may rest on me. That is why, for Christ's sake, I delight in weaknesses, in insults, in hardships, in persecutions, in difficulties. For when I am weak, then I am strong. (2 Corinthians 12:9–10)

Weakness doesn't have to mean defeat. It is my opportunity to experience God's power firsthand. Had I said yes to that one bite that first night of our vacation, there would have been more compromises. Compromise built upon compromise equals failure.

Instead, resisting temptation allowed promise upon promise to be built up in my heart, and that creates empowerment. This is God's power working through my weakness. I knew one day I would be empowered enough to take a couple of bites and walk away, but that day had not yet come.

I don't know what you might be struggling with today, but I can assure you that God is fair and just. There is a good reason we must face our temptations. The struggle to say no may be painful in the moment, but it is working out something magnificent within us.

For so long I've considered my struggles with weight a curse. I know I'm not alone in this. But, what if this battle with food is actually the very thing that, if brought under control, can lead us to a better understanding of God? What if we could actually get to the place where we thanked God for letting us face this battle because of the rich treasures we discovered on the battlefield?

My friend E. Titus summed up what I am discovering:

When I get all caught up in how unfair it is that my friend is skinny and doesn't have to work at it, how she can eat what she wants when she wants, and how much it stinks that I can't be like her, I remind myself that God didn't make me to be her. You see, He knew even before I was born that I could easily allow food to be an idol in my life, that I would go to food, instead of to Him, to fulfill my needs. And in His great wisdom, He created my body so that it would experience the consequences of such a choice, so that I would continually be drawn back into His arms. He wants me to come to Him for fulfillment, emotional healing, comfort—and if I could go to food for that and never gain an ounce, well then, what would I need God for?

There is such wisdom in my friend's perspective. Instead of parking her brain in a place where she constantly feels a struggle with food and weight issues, she's chosen a much healthier perspective.

The reality is, we all have things in our lives we have to learn to surrender, give up, sacrifice, turn away from. Think of that skinny girl in your life who you've watched eating whatever she wants. She may not struggle with her weight, but trust me, she has struggles. An anonymous comment on my blog gave vulnerable witness to this reality:

> I am one of the skinny girls, but don't mistake skinny for healthy. I battle depression and starvation, fight self-esteem issues from years of

verbal abuse, the list seems endless. Little is just an image. But being little doesn't make a person any more happy or faithful or joyful. The struggles are the same (or at least similar), just in a different-size package.

Life as a Christ follower will always be a learning process of depending less on our own strength and more on God's power. The Bible teaches that this "testing of [our] faith produces perseverance. Let perseverance finish its work so that [we] may be mature and complete, not lacking anything" (James 1:3–4).

Oh, sweet sisters, this truth should be the cry of our souls instead of Satan's lie that "it's not fair." Our taste buds make such empty claims to satisfy us, but only persevering with God will make us truly full, complete, not lacking anything.

Press on, sisters. Press on.

stinkin', rotten, horrible, no good day

I just don't have it in me to stick with this healthy eating thing," Amy said in utter exhaustion. Life had been spinning out of control in every area—troubled finances, a stressful marriage, struggling family members, and on and on. Because she couldn't control much about her life, Amy felt she could no longer limit her food choices. Food was her numbing drug of choice.

Forty-seven pounds later she sat sobbing on her bathroom floor. "What am I doing to myself?" She'd been carrying the weight of the world on her shoulders, and now everything was compounded by all the weight she'd added to her body.

As she crawled into bed, she glanced at the photo on her bedside table. There she was, nearly fifty pounds ago, smiling and hugging her husband. Where had that happy girl gone? Where had that happy couple gone? And when was the last time they'd even touched?

A deep knot of insecurity twisted in her gut at the

thought of her husband seeing her now. The only thing she wanted in that moment was the bag of Goldfish crackers and the half carton of Oreos sitting in her pantry.

My life is falling apart, and all I can think about right now is Goldfish and Oreos? It's a stinkin', rotten, horrible, no good day. Right now would be a really good time for the earth to swallow me up into a dark hole. Or for Jesus to come back. And speaking of Jesus, what an utter disappointment I must be.

Amy felt a dark depression slipping over her like a heavy blanket. A blanket so bleak and black she thought it might strangle the life out of her.

Ever been there? I have. Isn't it just like Satan to make us think we have to have something to comfort us, fill us, satisfy us, only to be haunted by the consequences of this comfort later?

Getting a Handle on Food During Hard Times

In the previous chapter, we talked about being tempted during times of celebration. But I think it's worth chatting about being tempted to overeat and make poor choices during times of struggle as well—when you just don't feel you have it in you to deny yourself unhealthy foods. Life is already denying you so much. For heaven's sake, everything you want seems out of reach, but these cookies are right here. And they will taste good. And no one has the right to say you can't have them. So there.

Obviously, I've been around this mountain or two or twenty-seven. But I love what my friend Ruth Graham says about traveling around the same mountain for far too long.

Either we can be victimized and become victims, or we can be victimized and rise above it. Often it is easier to play the victim than take off our masks and ask for help. We get comfortable with our victim status. It becomes our identity and is hard to give up. The Israelites often played the victim card, and I love what God finally tells them, "You have circled this mountain long enough. Now turn north" (Deuteronomy 2:3 NASB).

Turn north! It's time to move on! Self-pity, fear, pride, and negativity paralyze us. Taking off our masks takes courage, but if we don't do it, we will remain in our victim status and end up stunted.[5]

Or in this case overweight and unhealthy, further compounding our feelings of being victimized by our circumstances. So, what can we do when we don't have the energy, the fortitude, or the desire to eat healthy?

This is an important thing to tackle because if there is one thing I know about life, it will be dotted with hard times. We have to get a plan to realistically handle them and keep our compasses set to true north.

As Ruth stated, an important part of turning north is taking off our masks and asking for help.

For me, this starts with taking off my mask before the Lord and asking Him to help me find fulfillment in my relationship with Him. This means I have to admit there's a problem, and I really don't want to do that. Admitting I have a problem will likely require that I make changes, and changes are hard.

Food gives such an instant rush and tangible good feeling. It's so much easier to figure out how to get the short-term high of a cookie than it is to get a heart filled up and satisfied with God. I can drive to the store and fill my arms with any kind of cookies I want, but getting "filled up" with God during a particularly empty-feeling day doesn't seem as tangible or immediate.

I know I should pray. But I'm done with praying fake, plastic prayers when unhealthy snack options are calling to me and my resolve has worn as thin as a tissue. I have to have another prayer strategy. I have to find a way to be filled up and satisfied with God's love. And a few years ago, I found exactly what I needed—prayers where I don't speak at all.

Prayers Where I Don't Speak at All

I had been going through some stinkin', rotten, horrible, no good days and was at the absolute end of knowing what to pray. I'd slipped into a habit of praying circumst.___ oriented prayers where I'd list out every problem and ask God to please fix them. I even made suggestions for solutions in case my input could be useful. But nothing changed. Except my waistline.

In a huff one day, I sat down to pray and had absolutely no words. None. I sat there staring blankly. I had no suggestions. No solutions. I had nothing but quiet tears and some chocolate smeared across my upper lip. Eventually, God broke through my worn-out heart. A thought rushed through my mind and caught me off guard: *I know you want Me to change your circumstances, Lysa. But, right now I want to focus on changing you. Even perfect circumstances won't satisfy you like letting Me change the way you think.*

I didn't necessarily like what I heard, but at least I felt I was connecting with God. I hadn't felt that in a long time. And so, to keep that connection, I started making it a habit to sit quietly before the Lord.

Sometimes I cried. Sometimes I sat with a bad attitude. Sometimes I sat with a heart so heavy I wasn't sure I'd be able to carry on much longer. But as I sat, I pictured God sitting there with me. He was there already, and I eventually sensed that. I experienced what the apostle Paul taught: "The Spirit helps us in our weakness. We do not know what we ought to pray for, but the Spirit himself intercedes for us through wordless groans" (Romans 8:26).

As I sat in silence, the Spirit interceded with perfect prayers on my behalf. I didn't have to figure out *what* to pray or *how* to pray about this situation that seemed so consuming. I just had to be still and sit with the Lord. And during those sitting times, I started to discern changes I needed to make in response to my circumstances—none of which included using food for comfort.

I think a lot of us try to get filled up with things or people. In my book *Becoming More Than a Good Bible Study Girl*, I talked about how I walked around for years with a little heart-shaped cup, holding it out to other people and things, trying to find fulfillment. Some of us hold out our heart-shaped cup to food. Or expect relationships to fill up our insecurities. In other situations, it's wanting kids to be successful for a parent's own validation. Or, overspending the budget because that outfit would provide a temporary good feeling.

Whatever it is, if we are really going to stop circling the mountain and head north toward lasting changes, we have to empty ourselves of the lie that other people or things can ever fill our hearts to the full. Then we have to deliberately fill up on God's truths and stand secure in His love.

The more I do this, the less I find myself pulling out that little heart-shaped cup. I have to mentally replace the lies using some of my favorite verses to remind myself of just how filling God's love really is. Here are some examples of how I do that:

Old Lie: I need these Oreos. They will fill me up and taste so good.

New Truth: The thought that these Oreos
   me is a lie. They will taste good for just the few
   minutes it will take to eat them. Then that hollow feeling of guilt will rush in as soon as the
   chocolate high dissipates. Do I want to eat right
   now because I need nourishment or because I'm
   feeling empty emotionally or spiritually? If I
   truly need a snack right now, I am capable of
   choosing a healthier option.

Favorite Verse: "I pray that you, being rooted and
   established in love, may have power . . . to grasp
   how wide and long and high and deep is the
   love of Christ, and to know this love that sur-
   passes knowledge—that you may be filled to the
   measure of all the fullness of God" (Ephesians
   3:17–19).

Old Lie: I am such a failure with this healthy eating
   thing. Why sacrifice instant gratification now
   when I know eventually I'll just go back to my
   old habits anyhow?

New Truth: I am not a failure. I am a lavishly loved
   child of God. Part of my right as a child of God
   is to operate in a power beyond myself. The Holy
   Spirit is God's gift to me, so it is possible for me
   to use the self-control I've been given.

Favorite Verse: "See what great love the Father has
   lavished on us, that we should be called children
   of God! And that is what we are!" (1 John 3:1).

Old Lie: God seems so far away, and french fries are right around the corner at the drive-thru.

New Truth: French fries don't love me. And the only lasting thing I get from them is the cholesterol and cellulite they leave behind, which will just compound my frustration. God's love is here in this moment. His love is true and carries with it only positive residual effects.

Favorite Verse: "From everlasting to everlasting the LORD's love is with those who fear him" (Psalm 103:17).

This is just a start of replacing the lies and rationalizations with the truths of God's love. I encourage you to write out some old lies and new truths on your own. The process of stripping away old lies is hard and can produce raw feelings. That's why it's so crucial to have truths with which to replace them.

I pray we are all on this journey of replacing lies, embracing truth, and learning that food was never meant to fill the deepest places of our hearts reserved for God alone. Not on the good days. Not on the bad days. And not even on the stinkin', rotten, horrible, no good days. Jesus says, "See, I have placed before you an open door that no one can shut" (Revelation 3:8). May it be that we walk through that door, head north, and never look back.

12

curse of the skinny jeans

Once I reached my goal weight, I thought I'd never really have off-kilter days again.

Boy was I wrong.

It should have been a week of absolute rejoicing. I'd reached a major mile marker in my healthy eating journey—results. My skinny jeans fit. I was not only able to get them pulled up all the way and buttoned, but I could still breathe! Oh, yes ma'am, I could breathe and move and even sit down without the fear of bursting the seams.

Have you ever known this kind of crazy? Like most women, I had kept this pair of skinny jeans through many, many closet purges. All my other jeans from a size I hadn't seen in quite a while had long since been bagged up and taken to Goodwill. But this particular pair had been spared as a symbol of a promise I'd made to myself to one day lose the weight—again.

Every now and then I got out the jeans, crossed every possible finger and toe, and attempted to defy the odds by putting them on. I pulled and tugged and lay down on the floor to try and stretch this denim that must have shrunk in the dryer. I knew in my head it was not a case of laundry gone bad, but my heart was living in denial. With my refusal to make changes in my eating habits, the possibility of me ever wearing those jeans was nothing but wishful thinking.

Until now.

As I slipped the jeans on and buttoned them with ease, my smile could not be contained. I danced around my bedroom throwing my hands in the air. Sweet, sweet victory! I felt like I could take on the world. Until, just hours later, my world made me cry.

A hurtful email. A disrespectful attitude from one of my kids. A missed appointment. A messy house. A stressful situation at work. An unexpected bill. A dinner that was left basically untouched by my family. I found myself getting snappy, irritated with the sender of the email, on edge about the mess and stress, frustrated by that bill, and mad that no one liked my dinner.

How could I feel this way? I was wearing my skinny jeans, for heaven's sake! And I always thought that if only I could put on those skinny jeans, my whole world would fall into place and put a permanent smile on my face. Yet here I was, just hours later, falling prey to the same topsy-turvy stuff as before.

This is the curse of the skinny jeans. My body size is not tied to my happy. If my happy was missing when I was larger, it will still be missing when I get smaller.

Tying My Happy to the Wrong Things

Tying my happy to the wrong things is partially what caused my weight gain in the first place. There were too many experiences I enjoyed primarily because of the food that was attached to them. The movies were tied to popcorn. A birthday party was tied to cake. A ball game was tied to a hot dog. A morning meeting was tied to gourmet coffee. Watching TV was tied to chips. A summer outing was tied to ice cream. A winter outing was tied to hot chocolate.

Tying my happy to food, skinny jeans, or anything else sets me up for failure. Not to mention that once I slip on those skinny jeans, my elation is quickly marred by the fear of gaining back the weight.

I have to learn to attach my happy to the only eternal stability there is and remain there. Oh, the prayers I have prayed over and over and over for God to help me, stabilize me, and tie my happy only to Him. It's called learning to remain. Isaiah 55:8–12 illustrates so beautifully exactly what I'm talking about:

> "For my thoughts are not your
>   thoughts,
>   neither are your ways my ways,"
>   declares the LORD.
> "As the heavens are higher than the earth,
>   so are my ways higher than your ways

and my thoughts than your
thoughts.
As the rain and the snow
come down from heaven,
and do not return to it
without watering the earth
and making it bud and flourish,
so that it yields seed for the sower
and bread for the eater,
so is my word that goes out from my
mouth:
It will not return to me empty,
but will accomplish what I desire
and achieve the purpose for
which I sent it.
You will go out in joy
and be led forth in peace."

Did you catch how satisfying God's words are? They are compared to water that makes the earth bud and flourish. That's why Jesus' words in John 15 are so crucial for us to apply if we're ever going to have lasting joy.

Here's how Jesus described it:

As the Father has loved me, so have I loved you. Now remain in my love. If you keep my commands, you will remain in my love, just as I have kept my Father's commands and remain in his love. I have told you this so that my joy may be in you and that your joy may be complete. My command is this: Love each other as I have loved you. (vv. 9–12)

I'll admit, I've read these verses many times while nodding and saying, "Yeah, yeah, that's nice." But just recently, something new jumped out at me. We are taught to remain in God's love so that we won't tie our happy to anything but God. So that our joy will be complete.

Complete. As in not lacking anything. As in filled to the brink with joy. As in satisfied with a fullness we can't get any other way. Can you imagine how beautiful it would be to live as a complete person?

Incomplete people are difficult, demanding, and always in pursuit of that next thing. Incomplete people think that putting on their skinny jeans will right all their wrongs and fill up all their insecurities. Incomplete people quickly find out that their skinny jeans adjust nothing in their lives except the number on the tag.

Incomplete people are desperate for others to notice their diet progress, but they quickly realize that compliments don't assure connection or intimacy. They are not more liked or accepted or welcomed in.

The bad news is, we're all incomplete people. The good news is, Jesus loves incomplete people. And He wants us to know we can have complete joy by being secure enough in His love to reach out and love other incomplete people.

Afternoon Acts of Kindness

I'll admit, loving incomplete people doesn't seem like the obvious path to joy. And it doesn't seem like an obvious topic to cover in a book on getting healthy. But stick with me here; you might be surprised.

Just the other day I was pondering some of those distressing emails I mentioned earlier, and I reached the conclusion that incomplete people are a trigger that make me want to eat. They are complicated and sensitive and messy in their reactions, with the potential to drain my resolve and make me grumpy.

The last thing I want to do when a person throws their incompleteness in my direction is love them. I'd rather grab a bag of Cheetos and rationalize how much a treat is in order right now. Then I want to sit on my couch and tell the air around me how much I love Cheetos and how much I dislike incomplete people.

But what if I could be courageous enough to act and react like a complete person—a Jesus girl who has His joy in her sustaining and directing her? Instead of looking at this incomplete person's offense, what if I could see the hurt that surely must be behind their messy reaction?

I pause. I don't reach for the Cheetos. I don't react harshly out of my own incompleteness. I don't wallow in my thoughts of how unfair and unkind this other person is. I choose to love instead. Quietly taking out a piece of stationery and responding with words of grace. Or crafting an email with a message of compassion.

Better yet, what if I were to do this every afternoon, even when I haven't had a run-in with an incomplete person but am just simply craving things I shouldn't eat? I've been trying this out lately and I love it. Afternoon acts of kindness are yet another unexpected but beautiful result of letting Jesus direct my healthy eating pursuits.

Each day I've been asking Jesus who in my life needs words of encouragement, and He always puts someone on my heart. So instead of filling my afternoons with thoughts of frustration toward others or tempting thoughts about food, I am filling my afternoons with His thoughts of love toward others. And this is a great place to be no matter if I'm wearing my skinny jeans or not.

After all, the ultimate goal of this journey isn't about me becoming a smaller-sized person but about me craving Jesus and His truths as the ultimate filler of my heart. We are to remain in this healthy perspective. Let His thoughts be our thoughts. Remain. Let His ways be our ways. Remain. Let His truths go to the depths of our hearts and produce good things in our lives. Remain. Approach this world full of fellow incomplete people with the joy of Jesus. Remain. See our skinny jeans as a fun reward, nothing more. Remain. And be led forth in peace because I've kept my happy tied only to Jesus. Remain.

13

overindulgence

———————

I didn't quite know what to think as my pastor walked
up to the podium with a bottle of wine and proceeded
to pour a glass. Seeing a bottle of wine on center stage in
a Bible Belt church just doesn't happen. Ever. We drink
grape juice for Communion.

He then asked us to stand for a reading of God's
Word, which was the passage in John 2 where Jesus turns
water into wine. The point of his sermon was to clear
away some cultural taboos about drinking wine so that we
could see what the Bible really says.

Of course, my pastor handled this teaching very
delicately. Those who are underage or who have issues
with alcohol and can't have a glass of wine without being
irresponsible should avoid it altogether. He also touched
on not being a stumbling block to those who struggle.
Whether or not to have a glass of wine with dinner was
not the point of the sermon; the point was to know what
the Bible says about issues we face every day and to apply
those scriptures to our lives appropriately.

———————

Then he shifted gears and turned his attention to food.

Now this really was a historic churchgoing day. Seeing wine in the sanctuary was shocking enough, but never have I heard a preacher talk about gluttony in church. And his point was brilliant. How can we wag our fingers in the direction of alcohol only to walk into the church-wide covered-dish buffet and stuff ourselves sick with fried, smothered, grossly caloric delights that buckle our paper plates and cause our stomachs to cry for antacids?

Overindulgence is overindulgence. Eating or drinking in excess is a sin. The Bible calls it gluttony.

The biblical teaching about this is clear. "Do not join those who drink too much wine or gorge themselves on meat, for drunkards and gluttons become poor, and drowsiness clothes them in rags" (Proverbs 23:20–21). Here's another: "A discerning son heeds instruction, but a companion of gluttons disgraces his father" (Proverbs 28:7).

I imagine you are wondering if we really need to go there with this gluttony thing. It's not exactly the most girlfriend-fun topic. But we have to go there, and let me tell you why. On the surface, it appears that all we're talking about is food and the amount we consume. In reality, there is a more serious issue at the root. Overstuffing ourselves with food or drink or getting wrapped up in the affections of an inappropriate relationship are all desperate attempts to silence the cries of a hungry soul.

A Soul Longing to Be Filled

A starved soul is like the vacuum cleaner my mother used when I was a child. It had a long metal tube that ravenously sucked up anything and everything set before it. It sucked up dust bunnies with the same furor as it did a ten-dollar bill. I know that one from experience.

Our souls have the same ravenous intensity. That's how God created us—with a longing to be filled. It's a longing God instilled to draw us into deep intimacy with Him. The psalmist expressed this longing as an intense thirst: "As the deer pants for streams of water, so my soul pants for you, my God. My soul thirsts for God, for the living God. When can I go and meet with God?" (Psalm 42:1–2).

If we fail to understand how to fill our souls with spiritual nourishment, we will forever be triggered to numb our longings with other temporary physical pleasures. When those pleasures are food, the resulting behavior is often referred to as "emotional eating." But this issue is bigger than emotions; it's really about spiritual deprivation.

I hardly think it ironic that I'm struggling even as I write these words. A situation in my life has wormed its way straight to the most vulnerable places in my heart. And when my heart is feeling vulnerable, my resolve can become vulnerable too.

We'll talk more about emotional emptiness in the next chapter. For now, let's focus on the triggers that come on hard days, when part of me says, "You deserve treats, Lysa. Just one day of eating whatever you want and as much as you want."

I've realized that when the desire for treats is triggered by difficult emotions, it's not really a desire for treats—it's a thinly veiled attempt at self-medication. And self-medicating with food even once triggers vicious cycles I must avoid.

It's also important to note that not all gluttony is caused by emotional responses. Sometimes we overindulge because we lack the self-control to say enough is enough. And it breaks my heart how often people in the church simply turn their heads the other way when it comes to this issue.

So, What Are We to Do?

A few years ago, the words *portion control* took on new meaning as I studied the book of Exodus and noted the curious emotional response God's people had after Moses led them out of slavery in Egypt. They'd just seen God do miracle after miracle to help them escape their captors, but they panicked when it came to food.

> In the desert the whole community grumbled against Moses and Aaron. The Israelites said to them, "If only we had died by the LORD's hand in

Egypt! There we sat around pots of meat and ate all the food we wanted, but you have brought us out into this desert to starve this entire assembly to death."

Then the LORD said to Moses, "I will rain down bread from heaven for you. The people are to go out each day and gather enough for that day. In this way I will test them and see whether they will follow my instructions." (16:2–4)

In other words, God planned to use the Israelites' food issues to teach them the valuable lesson of daily dependence on Him. How?

Each day the Israelites were to ask God for their portion of food. Then God would rain down exactly what they needed for nourishment. It was called *manna*, which I imagine was something like sweet, little, potato flakes. The Israelites were to go out each day and collect just enough for that one day.

They were never to gather up extra and build big storehouses of manna supplies. No, God wanted them to take only their portion for one day. The next day they would come to Him and again receive their daily portion. The only exception to this was the day before Sabbath, when they could gather a double portion so they wouldn't have to work on the holy day.

We would do well to apply this same process to our struggles. Each day God can be the perfect portion of everything we need—every longing we have, every desperate desire our souls cry out for. God will be our portion.

With this in mind, let's visit a few of the emotional struggles that can often trigger a gluttonous response in us.

A relationship comes to an end. Instead of grabbing a tub of ice cream, I ask, "God, will You be my portion of healing and companionship for this day? I hate this rejection and hurt. Sometimes I feel like the loneliness is going to swallow me alive. I can't deal with this on my own. Be my portion."

That big business deal falls through. Instead of ordering the pasta dish drowning in cream sauce at lunch, I pray, "God, I so desperately want comfort right now, and that pasta seems like it would be so comforting. Feeling like a failure makes me want to say, 'Who cares,' and eat whatever. Will You be my portion of comfort and strength and success in this moment?"

My kids are driving me crazy. Instead of wolfing down three pieces of chocolate cake, I pray, "God, I so desperately want to be a patient mom. I don't know if I can be a patient mom the rest of my life. But with Your portion of strength I can rely on You in this moment and try not to medicate my shortcomings with food."

Whatever the situation, I keep asking God to be my daily portion over and over. And one day I will find victory over those things instead of just looking back over a pile of tears and cake crumbs. Here's a biblical promise we can rely on:

> Because of the LORD's great love we
>> are not consumed,
>>> for his compassions never fail.
> They are new every morning;
>> great is your faithfulness.
> I say to myself, "The LORD is my
>> *portion*;
>>> therefore I will wait for him."
>
> (Lamentations 3:22–24, emphasis added)

Grasping the truth that God is our portion has the potential to transform more than just our eating habits; it can transform our responses to every aspect of our lives. Practicing God's portion control was crucial for the spiritual development of the Israelites, and it's crucial for our spiritual development as well. God doesn't mince words about His expectations or His promises:

> You shall have no foreign god
>> among you;
>>> you shall not worship any god
>>>> other than me.
> I am the LORD your God,
>> who brought you up out of
>>> Egypt.
> Open wide your mouth and I will
>> fill it.
>
> (Psalm 81:9–10)

Whether we are talking about food, wine, sex, shopping, or anything else with which we try to fill ourselves, nothing in this world can ever fill us like God's portion. Nothing else is unfailing and absolute. And I don't say all this with a quirky little smile, hoping it works. I shout it from the depths of my soul because I know it works, "for he satisfies the thirsty and fills the hungry with good things" (Psalm 107:9).

14

emotional emptiness

One pound of fat is equivalent to thirty-five hundred calories, which makes gaining or losing weight a pretty straightforward mathematical equation. In order to lose weight, we need to burn more calories than we consume so our stored fat is burned off as fuel.

While this is as true for me as the next person, there are things that make the prospect of losing weight a little more complicated for me. Somewhere behind all the math, a less measurable force is at work within me. It takes the form of emptiness or lack. As I trace my fingers across the timeline of my life, I can remember times when spiritual and emotional emptiness left me vulnerable. The shape of my lack was the absence of a biological father. It was as if someone held up my family photo and excised his form from our lives with laser-like precision.

There we were—my mom, my sister, and me—with a hole that extended way deeper than an excised photograph. All of him was gone. His face that should have looked upon his children with adoration. His arms that should have worked to provide for us. His feet that I should have been allowed to stand on while he danced me around the den. His mind that should have shared wisdom about why pet hamsters die and why boys sometimes break girls' hearts.

He took with him so much more than he ever could have imagined. Those few suitcases and plastic crates didn't just contain boxers, ties, old trophies, and dusty books. Somewhere in between his Old Spice and office files were shattered pieces of a little girl's heart.

Now, I'm not a big fan of pointing to hurts from my childhood and saying, "All my issues can be linked back to what other people did to me." At some point I realized that everyone has hurts from their past. And everyone has the choice either to let those hurts continue to damage them or to allow forgiveness to pave the way to more compassion toward others. But the reality of my dad's abandonment created some unhealthy habits that lingered in my life.

Emptiness has a way of demanding to be filled. And when I couldn't figure out how to fill what my heart was lacking, my stomach was more than willing to offer a few suggestions. Food became a comfort I could turn on and off like a faucet. It was easy. It was available. And somehow, each time my heart felt a little empty, my stomach picked up on the cues and suggested I feed it instead.

When I decided to get healthy with my eating, I started by praying a very simple prayer: "Unsettle me." During my unsettling process I became aware of how emotional emptiness is a trigger for my eating. Much of this emotional emptiness stemmed back to that little girl coming home from school and being told, "Your daddy's gone." That one event was so huge, so draining, that it caused me to fill my mind with only negative memories of my dad. In my mind, he never loved me at all.

And you know what? Maybe he didn't. But parking my mind only on negative thoughts about my dad left such a sadness in my heart when I thought about what never was.

Sometimes I could brush off this sadness with a little sigh and recitation of who I am in Christ. But other times it made me angry. And defensive. And hungry. And deeply unsatisfied.

I honestly never thought anything but sadness was possible with my dad. I'd reached out to him with a few phone calls and letters over the years, but no miraculous restoration ever took place. No beautiful ending where he suddenly knocks on my door and says, "I'm sorry." No long-lost note that finally made its way to me that read, "I have always loved you." Just unresolved hurt and this nagging feeling that his absence was partially due to me not being what he wished I would have been.

That's a heavy weight for a little girl to carry. That's a heavy weight even for us big girls.

Then one day God surprised me in the most unusual way. I'd been praying for God to make me aware of all those places I'd resigned as impossible to change. And while my dad still made no effort to connect with me, a sweet memory of him changed my dark perspective.

Several winters ago, my family and I traveled to Vermont where I woke up one morning to stare at what an overnight snowstorm brought us. I had never seen such snow in all my life. But what really caught my attention were the gigantic icicles hanging from the roof line. They were glorious.

As I stared out at them, suddenly a memory of my dad flashed across the screen of my mind.

I grew up in Florida, which meant no snow ever. But I remember praying for snow. Praying like a revival preacher at a tent meeting, I tell you.

One night the temperatures dropped surprisingly low and the weatherman called for a freeze, which was a rare thing in our area. How tragic there was no precipitation. It was the one night that snow might have been possible.

It broke my little snow bunny heart.

But the next morning I awoke to the most amazing sight: icicles everywhere. Gleaming, dripping, hanging, light-reflecting, glorious icicles were all over the trees in our backyard.

It was magical.

We were the only house on the block with this grand winter display. Because I was the only girl whose daddy thought to intentionally put sprinklers out on the one night it froze.

I don't know where this memory had been hiding.

But what a gift. Somewhere in the deep, mysterious, broken places of my dad's heart, there was an inkling of love.

And while this certainly doesn't solve all the complications of being abandoned by my dad, it gives me a healthy thought to dwell on where he's concerned—one of those good thoughts the Bible tells us to think about: "Whatever is true, whatever is noble, whatever is right, whatever is pure, whatever is lovely, whatever is admirable—if anything is excellent or praiseworthy—think about such things" (Philippians 4:8). I like to call this "parking my mind in a better spot."

It's so easy to park our minds in bad spots. But this is where pity parties are held, and we all know pity parties demand an abundance of high-calorie delights. Pity parties are also a cruel way to entertain, for they leave behind a deeper emptiness than we started with.

And there I would sit with a guilt-ridden mind, a bloated stomach, an empty heart, and a soul full of anger that my dad was continuing to hurt me even all these years later.

But this icicle memory gave me a new place to park. A place where I could pursue truth rather than chocolate. A place where lovely could be something besides nachos in the Taco Bell drive-thru. And excellent could be my victorious response of turning to habits such as prayer, reading Scripture, and exercising away my stress rather than snacking away my emptiness.

What about you? Do you have something from

your past that causes emotional emptiness? As a first step toward healing, can you think of one good thing from this past situation? Or maybe something good that has happened despite the pain from the event? If not, ask God to give you some good places to park your mind. Then, try walking through the following exercise based on Philippians 4:8. Here's how I did this with the emptiness I felt about my dad:

Whatever is true: My dad was broken. Only broken daddies leave their children. This isn't a reflection of me. It's simply a sad reflection of the choices he made. But it's also true that he had to reach past his brokenness that one night to set up the sprinklers for his little girl. And as small as this one act is, it was an act of love.

Whatever is noble: I don't have to live as the child of a broken parent the rest of my life. I can live as a daughter of the King of kings who not only wants me but has promised to never, ever leave me. As a matter of fact, the Bible promises me, "The Lord is near" (Philippians 4:5). And the Lord was near the night of sprinklers. Though my dad professed to be an atheist, I'm convinced Jesus broke through his tough exterior that night and was near to him. Even if he didn't receive Jesus, my dad was near enough one night to see how beautiful love can be. I hope Dad remembers.

Whatever is right: Everything right and good in this life has God's touch on it. It makes me smile to think there must have been two sets of fingerprints on that rusty yellow sprinkler that night. My biological daddy set it up and turned it on. But my heavenly Daddy made sure the sprinkler was positioned just right to form icicles that froze the trees and warmed my heart.

Whatever is pure: God has set eternity in the heart of every human being (Ecclesiastes 3:11). So, even with all the darkness that seemed to surround my dad, some pure light of selflessness broke through and gave evidence of something good working within him. Warmth on a cold night. Purity in the midst of messy sin, broken hearts, and tainted lives.

Whatever is lovely: God can take ugly and build lovely from it. From the dust of the earth, He formed human beings. He healed a blind man by rubbing mud on the ailing man's eyes. That is a lovely quality about God. That lovely spilled over and helped my dad think of icicles. And in a backyard that never saw games of catch, a treehouse, or father-daughter talks, there was once a glorious display of lovely that only we had.

Whatever is admirable, excellent, or praiseworthy: I wouldn't say my dad was admirable, excellent, or praise-worthy. But then again, maybe I should. Maybe like the icicles, there are other memories long forgotten and covered over by the darkness of his cruel departure.

In the end, my Lord has taken those shattered pieces of my heart and removed them from the boxes my dad carried away that awful day. Piece by piece, God has created a mosaic in my heart—one of restoration, healing, and compassion. I am the person I am today in part because of the hurt of being left behind by my dad. I wouldn't have chosen that piece of my mosaic, but how good of God to place right beside the hurt a clear piece of glass shaped like those warm icicles from so long ago. A memory I can think on. A memory that is true, noble, right, pure, lovely, admirable, excellent, and praiseworthy. And filling.

I realize what I've written here is but a first step in this process. Often these issues are big and complicated and a bit like peeling back the layers of an onion.

If you need more help, be honest with yourself and seek out a good Christian counselor. Often churches can recommend counselors in your area who base their advice on biblical truths. I wouldn't be where I am today without asking counselors to speak truth into my life.

But for today, finding a gentle memory in the midst of a mess is a good start. A really good start. One worth looking for.

So, Dad, should you ever stumble upon these words, I pray you remember the night of the icicle wonder. For it is a common thread of hope that ties two very distant hearts together.

And that makes me smile.

15

the demon in the chips poster

In the last few chapters, we've been talking about replacing the old go-to scripts of rationalization with truth. Maybe I'm the only crazy dieter full of rationalizations, but here's another one we must address: "If no one sees you, then the calories don't count."

I know this makes absolutely no logical sense. But, girlfriend, sneaking when no one else is looking will absolutely kill a healthy eating plan. So, when I hear this rationalization playing out in my head, I don't try to replace it with a go-to script. Instead, I flee. I have to remove myself from the vicinity of the temptation.

Remember, this isn't just a battle in the physical and mental realm. This battle is spiritual as well. Satan wants us to sneak things in secret. Things hidden and done in secret clues in the father of darkness to our weaknesses and opens the door for him to assault us with targeted schemes. That's why the apostle Paul wrote, "Be strong in

---

the Lord and in his mighty power. Put on the full armor of God, so that you can take your stand against the devil's schemes" (Ephesians 6:10–11).

Here's how pastor and author Chip Ingram characterized Satan's schemes:

> They are orchestrated in order to tempt us, deceive us, draw us away from God, fill our hearts with half-truths and untruths, and lure us into pursuing good things in the wrong way, at the wrong time, or with the wrong person. The English word *strategies* is derived from the Greek word Paul uses that is translated "schemes." That means our temptations are not random. . . . The lies we hear, the conflicts we have with others, the cravings that consume us when we are at our weakest points—they are all part of a plan to make us casualties in the invisible war. They are organized, below-the-belt assaults designed to neutralize the very people God has filled with his awesome power.[6]

Did you catch what Chip included in his list of Satan's specific schemes? *Cravings that consume us when we are at our weakest points.* Yet we must remember we hold a power greater than any craving we face.

Just the other night I faced one of my fiercest battles with this.

I had a busy day and decided to grab take-out at one of my favorite restaurants on my way home. I ordered grilled fish and steamed broccoli. Pleased with my choice and my self-discipline, I proceeded to the pickup area. That's when the assault started.

A giant poster of the best chips and salsa you've ever seen was hanging over the take-out register. The girl behind the counter was trying to ask if I needed plastic-ware and to confirm my order.

Inside my brain a weak-willed woman started scream-ing, *No, my order is not correct! I need chips! Lots and lots of those chips!*

It was like those chips were dancing in front of me and singing the words from that eighties tune, "Don't you want me baby . . . don't you want me, ohhhhhh oh?"

I wanted to start reciting that old script in my head that would justify me right into a chips frenzy: *You've had such a hard day. You've been good for so long. Who would ever know? And if no one else knows, the calories don't really count, right? Plus, it's just one order of chips and salsa: Everything else you ordered is so healthy. Just do it this time and then be good for the next couple of days.*

But something else was tugging at my mind. Truth.

Lots of scriptures we've already covered sprang for-ward and started doing battle with the old script trying to lead me astray. I could feel the tension. Literally, as I stood there taking way too long to answer whether or not I needed a plastic fork, truth and lies were fighting for my attention. That's when it occurred to me: I held the power to determine who would win.

I held the power.

Not the chips.

And the power was to acknowledge that I'm not yet at a place where I can handle just a few chips. My brokenness cannot support that kind of freedom. Therefore, I had to flee. I had to remove myself from the source of temptation, and I had to do it immediately.

My hollow stare suddenly became an unwavering look of determination. "Yes, I do need a fork with this fish and broccoli." And I can picture the girl rolling her eyes as she bent down to get my fork, wondering what kind of fruit loop has to think for such an inappropriate amount of time about whether or not she needs a fork.

But I wasn't focused on her or her quizzical expression. Instead, I forced myself to focus on walking out that door.

As I drove home, one verse kept coming to mind: "They gave in to their craving . . . they put God to the test" (Psalm 106:14). By the time I got home and filled myself with the healthy fish and steamed broccoli, I realized I had no desire for chips and salsa. None. I was satisfied with my healthy choices.

What made the difference? Let's take a closer look at that verse in Psalms: "In the desert they gave in to their craving; in the wilderness they put God to the test."

The desert is a place of deprivation. In a deprived state we are much more likely to give in to things we shouldn't. I was really hungry when I walked into that restaurant. I was in a weakened state and faced with something that could instantly and easily fill me. That's what I call a danger zone.

Inside a danger zone the lies and rationalizations of the enemy sing so sweetly—alluring sights and smells coupled with salivating taste buds specifically arranged by the enemy for my destruction. This is the exact point at which I must start reciting truth, pack up my fish and broccoli, and flee. Deliberately flee.

I had to stop thinking about what I *shouldn't* have and park my mind on being thankful for what I *could* have. I could have delicious grilled fish and steamed broccoli. Food that is healthy and beneficial for my body.

We must embrace the boundaries of the healthy eating plan we choose. And we must affirm these boundaries as gifts from a God who cares about our health, not restrictive fences meant to keep us from enjoying life. Vulnerable, broken taste buds can't handle certain kinds of freedom. Boundaries keep us safe, not restricted.

I learned this through our sweet little dog, Chelsea. She is not the brightest bulb in the lamp. Though she has plenty of room to run and play inside our fenced-in yard, she is obsessed with trying to attack the tires crunching against our gravel drive whenever someone drives on our property. As a result, she had her second unfortunate encounter with a moving vehicle about the same time I started my healthy eating plan.

I wept like a baby when I saw her. But, other than a broken front leg, a severely scraped-up back leg, and a nose with half the flesh missing, she fared okay. Mercy.

The vet informed us that for her leg to properly heal, we'd have to keep her calm for three weeks. I asked if he could give her some nerve pills and throw a few in for me too. It would be a challenge to keep Chelsea still for three minutes. But three weeks?

Well, two weeks into the healing journey, all that stillness got the best of sweet Chelsea in the middle of the night. She decided she would punish me with a fit of whining, crying, and banging my closed bathroom door. She wanted out, and she wanted out now. She wanted to run and chase some unsuspecting night creature. She was sick of sacrificing her freedom.

To be honest, I wanted her to be able to run and chase a night creature too. But my love for this dog would not permit me to allow her to harm herself. Her brokenness couldn't handle that kind of freedom.

Not yet.

The truth behind Chelsea's brokenness struck me as quite applicable to myself as well. My brokenness couldn't handle freedom with food outside the boundaries of my plan.

Not yet.

Eventually, I will be able to add some things back into my diet in small quantities. But not yet.

My brokenness with food runs deep. Because it does,

my new healthy habits need time to run even deeper. Here are some of the healthy boundaries I have set to ensure success. I highly recommend reading through these often. They've proven to be really helpful for me to stay in a good place with my healthy habits.

- God has given me power over my food choices. I hold the power—not the food. If I'm not supposed to eat it, I won't put it in my mouth.
- I was made for more than being stuck in a vicious cycle of defeat. I was not made to be a victim of my poor choices. I was made to be a victorious child of God.
- When I am struggling and considering a compromise, I will force myself to think past this moment and ask myself, *How will I feel about this choice tomorrow morning?*
- If I'm in a situation where the temptation is overwhelming, I will have to choose to either remove the temptation or remove myself from the situation.
- When a special occasion rolls around, I can find ways to celebrate that don't involve blowing my healthy eating plan.
- Struggling with my weight isn't God's mean curse on me. Being overweight is an outside indication that internal changes are needed for my body to function properly and for me to feel well.
- I have these boundaries in place not for restriction

but to define the parameters of my freedom. My brokenness can't handle more freedom than this right now. And I'm good with that.

This battle is hard. Really hard. Whether you're at church staring at a covered-dish table heavy laden with all things breaded, fried, and smothered in cheese, or you're standing in a restaurant staring up at a chips-and-salsa poster, it can feel like a war is being waged in your head. So, I pray these boundaries help you like they've helped me.

Victory is possible, sisters, not by figuring out how to make this an easy process, but by choosing—over and over and over and over again—the absolute power available through God's truth.

16

why diets don't work

I have issues with infomercials. I do. I've ordered everything from grout cleaner to face powder to a meat griller that practically promised to grab the meat out of my fridge and cook it with no effort on my part.

However, no infomercials grab my attention quite like diet ones. With big promises and little sacrifice, you, too, can be a size smaller by this afternoon. And while everything in my brain screams, *It's a scam!* something in my heart says, *But maybe this one is the sure thing.*

Maybe this one really will make me feel so full I can eat three peas and half a chicken breast and be satisfied until dinner. Maybe this one really will block every bit of fat I consume from being absorbed in my body, thus allowing me to eat, eat, eat, without gaining, gaining, gaining.

In the end, my rational mind helps my wishful-thinking taste buds put the phone down, slip my credit card back into my wallet, and make peace with reality. There are no quick fixes.

But I have to hand it to these infomercial people.

They've figured out a way to tap into the harsh reality of why diets fail—we get tired of sacrificing and our self-effort wears thin.

I'm Not on a Diet

Recently, I was walking through the Chicago airport with some apple slices in my purse for a snack. I was perfectly happy with my apple until I walked past a smell that grabbed me by the collar, got right in my face, and said, "Don't you know how much happier I can make you?" A shop called Nuts on Clark had just made a fresh batch of caramel popcorn.

I love caramel popcorn. And I could easily rationalize purchasing some: I can't get this brand in North Carolina. It could be my special Chicago treat. Lots of other people were getting it.

Really, I could have gotten the popcorn, eaten a few handfuls and saved the rest for my kids, and been perfectly fine with my little diet cheat. The problem is, I'm not on a diet.

Diets don't work for me. I seem to be able to sacrifice for a season, and then I get tired of sacrificing. I hit my goal weight and then slowly slip into old habits. The weight creeps back on, and I feel like a failure.

So, I'm not on a diet. I'm on a journey with Jesus to learn the fine art of self-discipline for the purpose of holiness. And today I'd decided ahead of time I would have apple slices for a snack.

Deciding ahead of time what I will and will not eat is a crucial part of this journey. I also try to plan my meals right after breakfast, when I'm feeling full and satisfied. Deciding in advance keeps my thinking and planning rational and on track. The absolute worst time for me to decide is when I've waited until I'm feeling very hungry. At that point my body is screaming for something quick, and usually quick things come in a full variety of unhealthy temptations.

Here's a biblical perspective on temptation: "If you think you are standing strong, be careful not to fall. The temptations in your life are no different from what others experience. And God is faithful. He will not allow the temptation to be more than you can stand. When you are tempted, he will show you a way out so that you can endure" (1 Corinthians 10:12–13 NLT). The way out the Lord provides for me is deciding in advance what I will and will not have each day.

Verse 14 of this same chapter goes on to say, "Therefore, my dear friends, flee from idolatry" (NIV). Oh, how this verse points a finger straight at my issues with food and says, "This is exactly why this has to be a spiritual journey and not a temporary diet."

Expecting anything outside the will of God to satisfy us is idolatry. Nutrition, which is food's intended purpose, means consuming proper portions of healthy choices that enable our bodies to function properly. Idolatry, in the case of food, means consuming ill-sized portions and making unhealthy choices because we feel we deserve it or need it to feel better.

Now, hear me on this. We aren't to flee food. We need food. But we are to flee the control food can have over our lives. If we flee from the pattern of idolizing food and depending on food to make us feel emotionally better, we will be able to see more clearly the way out that God promises when we are tempted.

Two Elephants in the Room

As we're talking about those feelings of deserving or needing certain foods to get by, I think it quite appropriate to address two elephants in the room.

Elephant 1: "Don't tell me I have to give up all treats for all time."

I'm not saying we have to give up all treats for all time. When I was working toward getting to a healthy weight, I did give up all sugar and starchy carbs for a season. When I reached my goal weight, I added some things back to my eating but did so very carefully. Note the words *some* and *carefully*.

Now that I'm at my goal weight, if I were to decide in advance to have popcorn at the movies, then I would have a small popcorn (no butter). For the next several days

I would be more careful with my healthy eating regimen and take a pass on adding any treats.

Though this journey isn't all about weight loss, weight is a measure of whether or not we're making healthy choices. What I've experienced in previous weight-loss attempts is that prolonged success is really difficult.

I can't go back to my old habits of thinking I deserve a special treat every day. The realities of diet failure speak loudly and clearly that returning to old habits will cause the weight I've lost to return as well.

That leads me to the second elephant in the room.

Elephant 2: "I don't think this sounds like a spiritual journey. This sounds like a legalistic approach to eating."

Please hear my heart on this. I am writing this book as an invitation to consider the freedom found when we bring one of our most basic needs—food—before the Lord and allow Him to guide and guard us in this area.

We *do* need a healthy eating plan. But we must have a depth of restraint that can only come from making this a spiritual growth journey. The apostle Paul addressed this issue:

> Since you died with Christ to the basic principles of this world, why, as though you still belonged to it, do you submit to its rules: "Do not handle! Do not taste! Do not touch!"? These are all destined to perish with use, because they

are based on human commands and teachings. Such regulations indeed have an appearance of wisdom, with their self-imposed worship, their false humility and their harsh treatment of the body, but they lack any value in restraining sensual indulgence. (Colossians 2:20–23)

Pastor Ray Stedman commented on these verses:

A legalist looks at life and says, "Everything is wrong unless you can prove by the Bible that it is right. Therefore, we must have nothing to do with anything that the Bible does not say is right." That reduces life to a very narrow range of activity. But the biblical Christian looks at life and says, "Everything is right! God has given us a world to enjoy and live in. Everything is right, unless the Bible specifically says it is wrong." Some things are wrong; they are harmful and dangerous. Adultery is always wrong. So is fornication. Sexual promiscuity is wrong. Lying and stealing are wrong. These things are never right. But there is so much that is left open to us. If we are willing to obey God in the areas that he designates as harmful and dangerous, then we have the rest of life to enter into company with a Savior who loves us, and who guides and guards us in our walk with him.[7]

I especially love that last sentence. Entering into company with my Savior is indeed what I must do for this journey to be successful and long-lasting. It's the component that all my previous diets were missing.

Even the medical community is starting to pick up on the crucial role of spiritual commitment. Dr. Floyd Chilton, a physiologist who teaches at Wake Forest University School of Medicine, put it this way:

> Your willpower is in constant battle with your genes and your calorie-excessive environment. Often your best efforts are no match for your genes and environment. . . . Willpower alone is not enough to bring about this change; start by realizing that you cannot do this alone. If you are a person of faith, use that connection to help you change.[8]

God created us and told us to be faithful with the bodies we've been given. The Holy Spirit empowers us to make lasting change. And Jesus lovingly guides and guards us as we walk with Him, moment by moment, choice by choice, day by day.

And that's a plan with a promise no infomercial can ever offer!

things lost, better things gained

While we've already stated we don't have to give up all treats for all time, we will have to turn from some foods forever.

This turning is part courageous sacrifice and part utter repentance. And though the words *sacrifice* and *repentance* used to speak bitter-tasting hardship to my soul, they are speaking something else now. Something I've honestly grown to love. Victory.

But victory won't last for long if I start resisting and disliking its essential requirements of sacrifice and repentance.

I'm at my goal weight and in the most dangerous place for a dieting success story. It's time to celebrate— invite all those foods we've missed so much to a little welcome-home party, right? But we can't welcome home the missed foods without welcoming back all the calories, fat grams, cholesterol, sugars, and addictive additives.

The interesting thing about these "guests" is that they send out signals to our brains begging us to party with them again and again and again. A little welcome-home party becomes a reinvitation to be roommates, which spells disaster for what we hoped might be lifestyle changes.

For me, even little compromises with unhealthy cravings can quickly pave the road for an all-out reversal of my progress. And this is no longer just a personal revelation; science proves it. In a study published by *Science News*, researchers found junk food to be measurably addictive in lab rats:

> After just five days on the junk food diet, rats showed "profound reductions" in the sensitivity of their brains' pleasure centers, suggesting that the animals quickly became habituated to the food. As a result, the rats ate more food to get the same amount of pleasure. Just as heroin addicts require more and more of the drug to feel good, rats needed more and more of the junk food. "They lose control," [one of the researchers] says. "This is the hallmark of addiction."[9]

Other studies I read talked about the effect of certain sugary foods that turn off the body's ability to feel full.

It's really difficult for a chips-and-chocolate girl to uninvite foods to her party that have been regulars for years. And it's even more difficult to reconcile that they aren't my friends. Some can be casual acquaintances on a very limited level, but others need to be banished for good.

Only you can determine which is which.

A verse we've touched on before in this journey is worth repeating here: " 'Everything is permissible for me'—but not everything is beneficial. . . . I will not be mastered by anything" (1 Corinthians 6:12). Most people associate this verse only with sexual sins. However, the very next verse deals with food: " 'Food for the stomach and the stomach for food, and God will destroy them both' " (v. 13).

Talk about things that make a girl go *hmmm*. The commentary in my Bible remarks about these verses: "Some actions are not sinful in themselves, but they are not appropriate because they can control our lives and lead us away from God."[10]

Food is not the enemy. Satan is. And his strategic plan is to render us ineffective or at least sluggish for the cause of Christ. When we're stuck in issues of the flesh, it's really hard to passionately follow hard after God. So, lest we start mourning what will be lost, we must celebrate all that's being gained through this process.

What if this whole journey of getting healthy could be more about what we're in the process of gaining than what we're losing? In the midst of losing chips and chocolate, there are things to be gained. Things that unleash my weighted-down soul, reinflate my defeated attitude, and set loose a hope that maybe, just maybe, *I can*.

I can is a powerful little twist for a girl feeling deprived.

I can helps me walk into a dinner party and find the conversation more appealing than the buffet.

I can helps me stay on the perimeter of the grocery store where the fresher, healthier selections abound.

Today at lunch I threw away most of the sweet potato biscuit that came with my salad entrée. I'd taken a pinch off the side, enjoyed it immensely, and decided eating the rest would have been overdoing it. While tossing it, I smiled and said to myself, *This isn't a sign that I'm being deprived. This is a sacrifice I'm willing to make in order to gain something so much greater. This is the most empowering thing I can do in this moment!* I can. So, I did.

Whether we are at the beginning of our journey, in the middle, or in the danger zone of having just reached our weight-loss goals, focusing only on what we're giving up will make us feel constantly deprived. And deprivation leads to desperation, frustration, and failure. Instead, we have to focus on everything we're gaining through this process. And see the gains as more valuable than the losses.

Think of an old-fashioned scale. On one side, I place my chips and chocolate, and on the other side I place my newfound courage to say "I can." There's no comparison. My courage is so much more valuable and beautiful and empowering and lasting.

Chips and chocolate fill my mouth for a few seconds with a salty and sugary delight that has no life in it. But courage fills my heart, mind, and soul with everything alive and possible and invigorating.

And courage invites me to take one of the hardest steps on a journey like this. Courage says, *Now that you've partially turned from your old habits by making the necessary sacrifices, it's time to fully turn by repenting.*

Of all things lost and gained, the courage to repent might just be the most significant for me.

As I finish writing this book, I'm smack dab in the middle of the holidays. So, please excuse me if you are reading this in the summer and feeling very far from all things bright and jingle bell-ish.

I sat down today to spend a few minutes reading my Bible and decided to read the Christmas story in Mark. Well, it appears that Mark believed in cutting to the chase.

There's no mention of a manger. No Mary and Joseph. No baby Jesus. No bright star or angels. No silent night. No holy night.

As a matter of fact, if Mark were the only Gospel where Jesus' entrance to this world was mentioned, Christmas would look vastly different.

There would be no gifts.

No Linus delivering the stellar line in the Charlie Brown Christmas special.

No lights shining so brightly.

What would there be? A wild-looking man named John the Baptist dressed in leather and camel hair, preparing the way for Jesus by preaching a message we don't typically hear at Christmas. A message that's rough around the edges and a little hard to swallow.

Repentance.

That one word sums up the beginnings of Christ's

story according to Mark: "And so John the Baptist appeared in the wilderness, preaching a baptism of repentance for the forgiveness of sins. The whole Judean countryside and all the people of Jerusalem went out to him [c]onfessing their sins" (1:4–5).

This is about the place in the sermon where I start hoping some people I know are really paying attention. *Thank You, Lord, for this message. You know so-and-so needs a full-out repentance revival . . .*

It's at that point Jesus whispers to me, *It's a message to you and you alone. You need this message, Lysa. I am calling you to repent. This is the way you need to prepare for Christmas in your heart this year.* "I will send my messenger ahead of you, who will prepare your way—a voice of one calling in the wilderness, 'Prepare the way for the Lord, make straight paths for him'" (Mark 1:2–3).

The girl who can be such a mess.

Hears the messenger calling for repentance.

And she whispers once again, "I'm sorry, Jesus. Forgive me. Heal me. Restore me. Those little places I excuse. Those same old things that trip me up. The pride that keeps me thinking it's someone else's fault. The busyness that makes me forget to stop and consider my ways, my thoughts, my actions. You, Messiah, are the best match for my mess."

I doubt this will ever be the most popular version of the Christmas story, but for me this year it's a perfect place for this former chips-and-chocolate girl to complete this part of the journey. Not complete as in *I'm finished* so much as *I'm now perfectly prepared to carry on from here.*

Indeed, this has been one of the best spiritual journeys of my life. A significant, satisfying spiritual journey with great physical benefits. I have learned so much. But probably one of the richest lessons has been realizing the amount of mental and spiritual energy I wasted for years just wishing things would change. All the while beating myself up for not having the discipline to make those changes.

No matter what issue you are currently dealing with, Jesus wants to help you with it. He really does. But you have to stop beating yourself up about it and stand in the place of repentance.

Instead of using my shortcomings against myself, I can hand them over to Jesus and let Him chisel my rough places. The grace-filled way that Jesus chisels is so vastly different from the way I beat on myself. My beatings are full of exaggerated lies that defeat. His chiseling is full of truth that sets me free.

Oh, what a difference.

Jesus doesn't compare.

Jesus doesn't condemn.

Jesus doesn't exaggerate.

He simply says, *Hey, I love you. Just as you are. But I love you too much to leave you stuck in this. So, let's fully turn from those things that are not beneficial for you.*

I like that about Jesus.

I like that a lot.

Dear Jesus,

I have finally found the courage to admit I've craved food more than You. I have wept over giving up food while hardly giving a thought to You giving Your life for my freedom. I've been bound up by feelings of helplessness. I've been angry that I have to deal with this weight issue and have been mad at You for allowing this to be one of my lots in life. I've made excuses. I've pointed fingers. I've relied on food for things it could never give me. I've lied to myself about the realities of why I gain weight. I've settled and excused and justified my issues. I've been enthralled by buttered bread while yawning through Your daily bread.

For all that, I am so sorry. These are not just little issues. These, for me, are sins—missing the mark of Your best for my life. With my whole heart, mind, and soul, I repent. I turn from the dieting mindset. I turn from what I must give up and weep no more. I remove my toe keeping open the door to my old habits, my old mindset, my old go-to scripts.

I choose freedom. I choose victory. I choose courage. And above all else, I choose You.
Amen.

live as an overcomer

I was standing in the grocery store checkout line recently, gazing at rack after rack of magazines that bombarded me with promises of the latest diet fads. This is such a strange thing, really. The store wants me to buy lots of food, especially the high-profit junk food items. But as I'm paying for my food, the grocery store makes me look at magazines full of models that obviously don't spend a lot of time eating junk food or Paula Deen recipes.

All the models were a version of thin I'll never know. And they looked absolutely stunning in outfits meant for someone who has no body secrets.

Or, maybe their Spanx work a lot better than mine and the graphic artist who airbrushed their cover shot was incredibly generous.

Regardless, I stood there and for the first time realized my mind wasn't racing with self-condemnation. I simply smiled. And I realized my victory isn't tied as much to the way I've changed physically as it is tied to the way I've overcome mentally and spiritually.

Yes, I've lost pounds and inches. But not being

weighted down mentally and spiritually by the constant feeling of defeat is the real victory.

This freedom is not tied to a person's size. There are painfully thin women weighted down spiritually and emotionally by feelings of defeat the same as women many sizes larger. I truly think that on some level most of us girls struggle with this whole "getting healthy" thing. After all, the very downfall of humanity happened around a circumstance where a woman was tempted with food.

We've seen throughout this journey that God doesn't just command us to have a healthy perspective on food, He also provides the help to achieve it. His Word holds the key for anyone wanting to overcome food issues, be they slight, severe, or anywhere in between. His truths perfectly direct us, guide us, and teach us. And He's proven true to His promises to save us:

> Some became fools through their
>   rebellious ways
>   and suffered affliction because
>   of their iniquities.
> They loathed all food
>   and drew near the gates of death.
> Then they cried to the LORD in their
>   trouble,
>   and he saved them from their
>   distress.

(Psalm 107:17–19)

While I can't say I was drawing near to the gates of death physically when I was struggling in this journey, I was drawing near to a complete sense of defeat, wondering if overcoming this haunting struggle was even remotely possible.

That's an awful place to be.

How precious of God to know and address so specifically a woman's struggle with food. Back up and read that psalm again.

How does He save them?

How does He save the person with issues like mine?

How does He save the anorexic girl who loathes all food?

How does He save the severely obese who truly are drawing near to the gates of death?

How does He save any of us who are acting foolish and rebellious?

The next verse of Psalm 107 gives the answer: "He sent out his word and healed them; he rescued them from the grave" (v. 20).

He sent forth His word, and His word healed them!

Jesus girls aren't made to get stuck in a state of defeat. We were made to walk on paths headed toward victory. Not starting Monday, but starting right now. This doesn't mean these paths won't be riddled with struggles we'll need to learn to overcome. They will. For lessons on overcoming are some of God's greatest and most enduring gifts.

Just the other day I found some of the most fascinating verses about overcoming in the book of Revelation. This is normally a book of the Bible around which I'm a little skittish; I feel like I should possess a degree of some sort before knocking on its door. But last week in church the pastor read a verse that intrigued me. I flipped to that verse and soon found myself intrigued with many verses.

This might be the verse that elicits the greatest excitement in my heart. "To him who overcomes, I will give the right to *eat* from the tree of life, which is in the paradise of God" (Revelation 2:7, emphasis added).

Isn't it thrilling to see that overcoming is possible? It is possible to be more than just one who *deals* with their struggles well. This verse says, to the one who *overcomes*! In other words, it's for those who find absolute victory in an area where they once knew nothing but defeat.

And there's a reward for pressing through our struggles all the way to absolute victory. How absolutely tickled I am to know that the reward for overcomers is that they are given the right to *eat*! Eating from the Tree of Life will be unlike any satisfaction we've ever known. And might I just note that because it specifically says this tree is located in paradise, we will be eating in heaven.

Oh, yes, we will.

This is why I smiled while standing in that grocery store checkout line last week. The circumstances were all the same. The magazines were still strategically placed to get my attention. The models were still airbrushed beyond reality. And I still had to buy food.

But my response to all these same circumstances changed because I have changed inside. I have found my "want to" physically, emotionally, and spiritually.

My healthy choices make me feel empowered, not deprived. My healthy go-to scripts come so naturally, they aren't rules I follow but the natural way I think about food. And I'm excited about this being my lifestyle. Truly excited.

I hope you are as well. I'll admit, I'm a little sad this book is coming to an end. I have enjoyed walking with you through this journey. But while the book is ending, living out its message is just beginning.

Dare to set your toes firmly on the pathway of victory you are meant to be on. Whether we're on the path toward victory or defeat is determined by the very next choice we make. Not the choices from yesterday. Not the choices made five minutes ago.

The next choice. Our very next choice. May it be that of an overcomer. An overcomer made to crave God alone.

healthy eating
go-to scripts

---

1. God has given me power over my food choices. I'm supposed to consume food. *Food isn't supposed to consume me.*

   > He said to me, "My grace is sufficient for you, for my power is made perfect in weakness." . . . For when I am weak, then I am strong. (2 Corinthians 12:9–10)

2. *I was made for more* than to be stuck in a vicious cycle of defeat.

   > You have circled this mountain long enough. Now turn north. (Deuteronomy 2:3 NASB)

3. When I'm considering a compromise, I will think past this moment and ask myself, *How will I feel about this choice tomorrow morning?*

   > Do you not know that your bodies are temples of the Holy Spirit, who is in you, whom you have received from God? You are not your own;

you were bought at a price. Therefore honor
God with your bodies. (1 Corinthians 6:19–20)

4. When tempted, I either *remove the temptation* or
   remove myself from the situation.

   If you think you are standing firm, be careful
   that you don't fall! No temptation has over-
   taken you except what is common to mankind.
   And God is faithful; he will not let you be
   tempted beyond what you can bear. But when
   you are tempted, he will also provide a way out
   so that you can endure it. Therefore, my dear
   friends, flee. (1 Corinthians 10:12–14)

5. When there's a special event, I can find *other ways to*
   celebrate rather than blowing my healthy eating plan.

   See, I have placed before you an open door
   that no one can shut. (Revelation 3:8)

6. *Struggling with my weight isn't God's mean curse on me,*
   but an outside indication that internal changes are
   needed for me to function and feel well.

   "Forget the former things;
        do not dwell on the past.
   See, I am doing a new thing! . . .
   I am making a way in the desert
        and streams in the wasteland."

                                    (Isaiah 43:18–19)

7. I have these boundaries in place *not for restriction* but to *define the parameters of my freedom.*

    > I am using an example from everyday life because of your human limitations. Just as you used to offer yourselves as slaves to impurity and to ever-increasing wickedness, so now offer yourselves as slaves to righteousness leading to holiness. (Romans 6:19)

notes

1. Dictionary.com, s.v. "craving," http://dictionary
   .reference.com/browse/craving.
2. Dictionary.com, s.v. "enlightened," http://
   dictionary.reference.com/browse/enlightened.
3. Used by permission of Karen Ehman. You can
   find this post on her delightful blog: "Defined by
   Obedience, Not by a Number (and a Giveaway!!),"
   Karen Ehman, October 28, 2009, http://
   karenehman.com/home/2009/10/28/defined-by
   -obedience-not-by-a-number-and-a-giveaway/.
4. Ralph Waldo Emerson, quoted in Maddie Ruud,
   "Inspirational Quotes About Beauty–Body Image
   Quotes," HubPages, March 8, 2011, http://
   hubpages.com/hub/Quotes_on_Beauty.
5. Ruth Graham, *Fear Not Tomorrow, God Is Already
   There* (New York: Howard Books, 2009), 104–5.
6. Chip Ingram, *The Invisible War* (Grand Rapids:
   Baker, 2006), 27.
7. Ray Stedman, "The Things That Can Ruin Your
   Faith," message on Colossians 2:16–23 delivered

January 25, 1987, Ray Stedman Ministries (Sonora, CA), http://www.raystedman.org/new-testament /colossians/the-things-that-can-ruin-your-faith.

8. Floyd Chilton, quoted in "Help, I Can't Stop Eating," *US Airways Magazine*, June 2009, https:// nutrition.cals.arizona.edu/person/floyd-ski-chilton -phd.

9. Laura Sanders, "Junk Food Turns Rats into Addicts," *Science News*, October 21, 2009, https://www .sciencenews.org/article/junk-food-turns-rats-addicts.

10. "1 Corinthians," in *NIV Life Application Study Bible* (Grand Rapids: Zondervan, 2004), 2070n6:12.

about the author

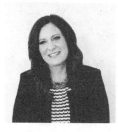

Photograph by Kelsie McGarty

Lysa TerKeurst is the president of Proverbs 31 Ministries and the #1 *New York Times* bestselling author of *Forgiving What You Can't Forget, It's Not Supposed to Be This Way, Uninvited, The Best Yes,* and twenty-two other books. But to those who know her best, she's just a simple girl with a well-worn Bible who proclaims hope in the midst of good times and heartbreaking realities.

Lysa lives with her family in Charlotte, North Carolina. Connect with her on a daily basis and follow her speaking schedule:

Website: LysaTerKeurst.com
(Click on "events" to inquire about
having Lysa speak at your event.)
Facebook.com/OfficialLysa
Instagram: @LysaTerKeurst
Twitter: @LysaTerKeurst

If you enjoyed *I'll Start Again Monday*, equip yourself with additional resources for your healthy-eating journey at:

illstartagainmonday.com

About Proverbs 31 Ministries

Proverbs 31
MINISTRIES

Lysa TerKeurst is the president of Proverbs 31 Ministries, located in Charlotte, North Carolina.

If you were inspired by *I'll Start Again Monday* and desire to deepen your own personal relationship with Jesus Christ, we have just what you're looking for.

Proverbs 31 Ministries exists to be a trusted friend who will take you by the hand and walk by your side, leading you one step closer to the heart of God through:

Free *First 5* Bible study app
Free online daily devotions
Online Bible studies
Podcast
COMPEL Writer Training
She Speaks Conference
Books and other resources

Our desire is to help you to know the Truth and live the Truth. Because when you do, it changes everything.

For more information about Proverbs 31 Ministries, visit www.Proverbs31.org